NATURE AND TREATMENT OF ARTICULATION DISORDERS

NATURE AND TREATMENT OF ARTICULATION DISORDERS

By

JOHN P. JOHNSON, Ph.D.

*Associate Professor of Speech Pathology
Programs in Speech Pathology, Audiology
and Deaf Education
Lamar University, Beaumont, Texas*

With a Contribution by

Robert D. Moulton, Ph.D.

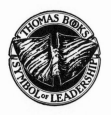

CHARLES C THOMAS · PUBLISHER
Springfield · Illinois · U.S.A.

Published and Distributed Throughout the World by
CHARLES C THOMAS • PUBLISHER
Bannerstone House
301-327 East Lawrence Avenue, Springfield, Illinois, U.S.A.

©*1980, by* CHARLES C THOMAS • PUBLISHER
ISBN 0-398-03983-6
Library of Congress Catalog Card Number: 79-21042

With THOMAS BOOKS careful attention is given to all details of manufacturing and design. It is the Publisher's desire to present books that are satisfactory as to their physical qualities and artistic possibilities and appropriate for their particular use. THOMAS BOOKS will be true to those laws of quality that assure a good name and good will.

Library of Congress Cataloging in Publication Data

Johnson, John P.
    Nature and treatment of articulation disorders.

    Bibliography: p.
    Includes index.
    1. Articulation disorders. I. Moulton, Robert D.,
joint author. II. Title. [DNLM: 1. Articulation
disorders. 2. Articulation disorders — Therapy.
WM475.3 J67n]
RC424.7J3   616.8'554   79-21042
ISBN 0-398-03983-6

Printed in the United States of America
C-1

to my wife
Barbara
and my three children
Michael, Scott, and Traci

PREFACE

THIS BOOK is designed as a comprehensive text on the nature and treatment of articulation disorders. It is primarily intended to serve as a text for undergraduate and graduate students majoring in speech pathology. However, it is hoped that it will also provide a valuable reference source and clinical update for the practicing speech pathologist.

Recent advances in our knowledge of the nature of normal and defective articulation have had a marked influence on the practice of speech pathology. During the past two decades the profession has witnessed and participated in the evolution of modern phonological theory. During the same period there has been a proliferation in the growth of our understanding of the central organization and motor control of speech. Research has increased our knowledge of articulatory growth and development and has, at least tentatively, identified some of the variables associated with articulation learning.

These developments have had significant impact upon clinical management practices and have rendered many of the older texts on the subject obsolete. Although a number of excellent new books have emerged in recent years, they have typically focused on a single aspect of articulation and are too unidimensional to be considered as a comprehensive text or reference on the subject. This has provided the impetus for the present writing.

The purpose of the book is to provide students of speech pathology with a single reference source that reviews many of the relevant contributions of the past, summarizes meaningful, contemporary research findings, and discusses both in the pragmatic light of clinical management considerations.

Unquestionably, some readers may feel that certain aspects have been slighted while others may contend that some of the sections are presented with too much attention to detail. For those in the first category, I have attempted to include at the end of each chapter an adequate bibliography for supplementary reading. For those who may fall into the second category, I can only say that every book necessarily reflects the biases of its author and ask that the reader be tolerant of mine.

The first four chapters are concerned with the nature and development of both normal and defective articulation and provide the foundation for the subsequent discussion of clinical management in Chapters 5 through 8. The focus is on articulation as a multifaceted process. Normal articulatory behavior requires the development and integration of a number of underlying systems. Therefore, the term *articulation disorder* is viewed by the author as a generic classification, not a diagnosis. Specification of disorder type is required. In recent years it has become obvious that articulation disorders involve more than a simple inability to correctly produce speech sounds. Disorders may reflect a deviant phonological pattern, difficulty in the central encoding of speech, deficits affecting the phonetic, articulomotor aspects of production, or a combination of these. It is the responsibility of the clinical speech pathologist to identify the disorder type and associated variables in each individual case and, based upon this information, to select and implement an appropriate therapy program. The task is frequently a difficult one. The book will hopefully make the process easier.

It is not uncommon to hear students in clinical practice speak of "simple articulation cases." In response, I suggest that the only thing simple about articulation disorders is the mind that labels them so.

J.P.J.

Acknowledgments

T HE WRITING OF A BOOK is a difficult process and, without the assistance and cooperation of significant others, represents an almost impossible endeavor. First and foremost, I would like to extend my appreciation to Doctor Robert Moulton for writing Chapter 8. His experience and expertise in deaf education are manifest in the chapter, and his contribution to the book is of major importance. Further, his encouragement and administrative support are gratefully acknowledged. Appreciation is also extended to Mrs. Betty Winney, Doctor Robert Achilles, and Doctor Olen Pederson for reviewing portions of the manuscript and providing valuable suggestions and insights. Similarly, I am indebted to my many students for their critical reviews and constructive comments. Special acknowledgments go to two of my former teachers, Doctor Sam Faircloth, for originally introducing me to the subject, and Doctor Ron Sommers, for providing me with the guidance and opportunity for in-depth study. Finally, appreciation is extended to Paula Adams and Diane Shaffer for typing and assisting with the manuscript.

Contents

NATURE AND TREATMENT OF ARTICULATION DISORDERS

CHAPTER 1

The Nature of Articulation

COARTICULATION AND THE MOTOR CONTROL OF SPEECH

FOR YEARS it has been the practice of speech pathologists to identify the sounds that clients misarticulate and then to work on correcting them in isolation, in syllables, in words, etc., progressing from one level to the next as proficiency is achieved. While this procedure may eventually result in improvement, it is certainly inconsistent with the nature of speech articulation and is not congruent with the original and natural processes of articulation learning.

Unlike letters printed out by a typewriter, speech sounds are not produced separately and then strung together to form syllables, words, and higher level linguistic units. If this were the case it would be nearly impossible for an individual to maintain even an average rate of speech (approximately twelve speech sounds per second). Our ability to start and stop the movements of our articulators (diadochokinesis) is limited. Rapid rates of speech of eighteen to twenty speech sounds per second would literally be impossible if we produced sounds as individual, separate units. Further, the ability of the listener to discern individual acoustic units breaks down at approximately eighteen per second. That is, if we were to tap on a table at a rate greater than eighteen times per second the average listener would no longer be able to identify individual taps and would, instead, perceive a low frequency tone. Thus, if speech sounds were individually produced, rapid rates of speech would challenge the resolving power of the ear, and speech would sound like a low frequency buzz. This is obviously not the case.

Speech sounds are not produced autonomously. They share space and time with their neighbors. They overlap one another in ongoing connected speech. Certain characteristics of previous and upcoming sounds in a connected speech sequence will appear in the sound being produced. The generic term used to describe this phenomenon is *assimilation*. However, when describing or identifying the overlapping movements of the articulators, which provide the underpinnings for observable assimilative effects, speech pathologists generally use the term *coarticulation*. The popularity of the term can probably be attributed to the fact that coarticulation refers directly to the articulomotor bases of speech.

The fact of coarticulation, i.e. that neighboring sounds affect each other, has long been known. In 1933, Bloomfield stressed the point that the positions of the articulators for a given speech sound were altered somewhat to be more compatible with those of neighboring sounds. Spriestersbach and Curtis, in 1951, demonstrated that consonants misarticulated as singletons were frequently articulated correctly when occurring as the second element of a blend. In 1954, Curtis demonstrated that overlapping articulatory movements in connected speech segments produced significant observable variations in the acoustic pattern. This study revealed that when individual speech sounds were articulated in a connected manner, the acoustic end product was not simply the combination or sum of the acoustic characteristics of the two individual sounds, but rather a new acoustic pattern. Based on these and other similar early investigations and stressing the dynamic, overlapping nature of speech, McDonald (1964) defines articulation as "a process consisting of a series of overlapping, ballistic movements which place varying degrees of obstruction in the way of the outgoing airstream and simultaneously modify the size, shape and coupling of the resonating cavities" (p. 87).

It is not unusual for students who have completed their first course in phonetics to think of speech sounds in static, fixed terms, such as place of articulation. However, it is apparent that production involves multiple movements of more than a single articulator. McDonald's definition uses the terms "ballistic movements" that "simultaneously modify" the size and shape of the vocal tract. The production of a given speech sound involves the simultaneous movement of a number of the articulators with certain *trajectories* and multiple *targets*. For example, the production of the sound /b/ requires a progressively approximating movement of the lips with the target of bilabial contact, posterior-superior movement of the velum with the target of velopharyngeal contact, medial movement of the vocal folds with the target of adduction for voicing, and so on. Obviously, these movements are occurring simultaneously.

The amount of influence neighboring sounds have on one another, i.e. the magnitude of observable coarticulation, is therefore contingent upon the degree of compatibility among the respective articulator trajectories and target values of each sound and the reciprocal adjustments made. In addition to phonetic context, rate of speech and differential stress may also affect the magnitude of coarticulation. Thus, the trajectory of a given articulator may be altered and will vary according to the trajectory targets for preceding and upcoming speech sounds and, possibly to a lesser extent, according to speech rate and stress requirements. As a result, the ideal target may not be hit but only approximated in ongoing speech. This is referred to as articulatory (target) *undershoot/overshoot*.

When considering the coarticulation effects of phonetic context we can identify two possible sources of influence: sounds that precede and sounds that follow the sound being produced. When the articulator trajectories-targets of a preceding sound overlap with and influence those of the sound being produced, it is referred to as left to right or *backward* coarticulation. For example, when the /s/ sound follows a voiced sound, such as in the word "boys," it is frequently voiced and produced as /z/. On the other hand, when it follows a voiceless sound, such as in the word "beats," it is voiceless. The /k/ sound is produced more posteriorly in the word "look" than in the word "leak" due to the influence of the preceding vowels. Similarly, consonants and vowels following the consonants /m/ and /n/ are generally more nasalized than those following nonnasal consonants.

When upcoming sounds influence the trajectories and targets of the sound being produced, it is referred to as right to left or *forward* coarticulation. It has also been referred to as anticipatory coarticulation since it is obvious that articulatory adjustments must occur in anticipation of the articulomotor characteristics of an upcoming, yet to be produced sound. For example, in the word "ask," the tongue movement for /k/ begins before the completion of the tongue movement for /s/. If the reader will slightly exaggerate and prolong the word, you should be able to feel the front to back movement of the tongue during the production of /s/ in anticipation of the tongue target for /k/.

In the word "puptent" the two /p/ sounds are obviously produced differently. The initial /p/ is aspirated as it releases into the vowel while the second /p/ is unreleased as it coarticulates with /t/. In the word "stool," lip-rounding in anticipation of the vowel begins with /s/ and makes it physiologically and acoustically different than the /s/ in the word "steel" or other phonetic contexts. In the word "treatment," while the tongue is in contact with the alveolar ridge for the production of the second /t/, the lips are closing, the vocal folds are adducting, and the velum is lowering in anticipation of the upcoming /m/ sound.

This last example points out the fact that coarticulation involves more than a single articulator. In addition, both backward and forward coarticulation effects may be observed in a given phonetic environment and may be seen to span several sounds. In a 1968 study by Daniloff and Moll, forward coarticulation was found to span four consonants without regard for syllable or word boundaries.

From the above it should be obvious that coarticulation and phonetic contexts greatly influence articulatory accuracy and the extent to which the targets for a given speech sound are achieved. Clinical speech pathologists are well aware of the fact that children who misarticulate speech sounds are frequently inconsistent in their misarticulations. In fact, however, these children may be quite consistent in their error patterns, articulating the sound correctly in some phonetic contexts while missing the salient targets in others. For example, it seems reasonable to assume that a child might be able to produce the /s/ sound with greater accuracy when it follows or precedes a /t/ than in consonant or vowel contexts with more dissimilar tongue targets.

Coarticulation effects may allow for correct production in some contexts and result in incorrect production in others for clients with articulation defects; however, variation of this magnitude is typically not seen in normal speech production. Although all sounds are affected by phonetic context and, as a result of coarticulation, are produced somewhat differently, they are still recognized by the listener as belonging to a given speech sound class. Thus, even though the first and second /p/ sounds in the word "popcorn" are different, the listener nonetheless perceives both as members of the /p/ family.

Such a family is referred to as a phonemic group. A *phoneme* is an abstract categorization with certain core characteristics (stimulus values) that signal semantic reference. Even though the /p/ sounds in the above example are acoustically and physiologically different, their core characteristics are maintained to a sufficient degree that the listener is able to identify them as belonging to the phoneme /p/.

Variations that do not change one speech sound to another one (one phoneme to another phoneme) are referred to as *allophonic* variations in production. For example, the first and second /p/ sounds in the above example are allophones of the phoneme /p/. The first is aspirated and released while the second is unaspirated and unreleased.

Depending on the language of the speaker-listener, some articulatory gestures are phonemic (signal a change in meaning) while others are allophonic. If we were to produce voicing on the /p/ it would become a /b/ and, thus, the gesture would be phonemic in nature. On the other hand it is obvious from the above example that aspiration as a part of a plosive is a nonphonemic, allophonic variation in English. Since all phonemes undergo some change in connected speech as the result of coarticulation and phonetic context, it is safe to say that we do not produce phonemes but rather allophones.

Considering the fact that there are an extremely large number of possible contexts for a given phoneme it is reasonable to conclude that there are an equally large number of allophones. Is it no wonder that children are frequently inconsistent in their misarticulations of a given phoneme? The fact is that children do not misarticulate and speech pathologists do not work on correcting a single phoneme at the production level. Rather, multiple allophones of a given phoneme may be defective, depending upon the *consistency* of the misarticulation.

Although speakers produce allophones, listeners apparently perceive phonemes. This phenomenon has been referred to as perceptual invariance or constancy in the face of rather substantial acoustic variation. This will be discussed in greater detail in the upcoming section on perception. However, it would seem that as listeners we are able to tolerate a good deal of variation in the acoustic signal and the way in which phonemes are produced and still recognize the pattern as a given phoneme. Allophonic variation, as indicated above, is partially a by-product of phonetic context and coarticulation effects. However, variation also occurs as the result of speaker differences. Even if the phonetic context is the same, allophones will vary as the result of differences in the size, shape, and timing characteristics of one speaker's speech mechanism as contrasted to that of another speaker. Speaker to speaker variation may also occur as the result of differences in dialect, stress, rate of speech, and early articulomotor (phonetic) learning influences. However, even though there are a number of sources of substantial allophonic variation, listeners are generally able to identify the target phoneme, given that the salient characteristics (distinctive features) are adequately represented. When the articulatory gestures and their corresponding acoustic correlates are missing or severely distorted or when the articulomotor variation results in an off-target phonemic change, we label it as a misarticulation. Consideration of a client's allophonic error pattern for a given phoneme is important to clinical management and will be discussed further in Chapters 5, 6, and 7.

Of equal importance, or perhaps potentially of greater importance than the above, would be an understanding of how speech is programmed for production purposes. What are the units of speech that are learned, stored, recalled when needed, and fed forward to the neuromotor system for execution? Are the input units to the motor system subphonemic articulatory gestures, phoneme in size, syllables, or perhaps larger in size? How are the units organized into appropriate combinatorial form? At present we do not have any definitive answers to these questions. However, research has provided us with interesting speculations and a few viable theories. Prior to discussing these, however, a brief verbal schematic of how speech is produced would seem to be warranted.

It is generally believed that an area of the cortex immediately surrounding the anterior third frontal convolution in the left hemisphere (Broca's Area) is a memory center for the motor movements of speech. As the developing child acquires an awareness of the correspondence between selected articulator movement patterns and the acoustic product, the information is stored and becomes available for future reference. As further development occurs, his available repertoire grows and his program (knowledge) of the motor patterns and sequencing needed to achieve a given speech segment eventually becomes complete. The first step in speech production would involve language formulation, an activity generally felt to occur in the temporal-parietal lobe regions of the cortex. In order for the language to be externally realized the linguistic units must be coded in terms of the neural commands that will be needed to innervate the speech mechanism musculature to produce the desired acoustic pattern. It is believed that the speech motor memory center provides this coding operation, translating or recoding the language units into neural commands.

This coding operation and the size and character of the neuromotor command units (input units) represent the topic of central concern to the present discussion. At any rate, once generated the neuromotor commands are relayed to the inferior portion of the "motor strip" (precentral gyrus) for neuromotor execution. This area of the cortex contains large motor neurons capable of initiating neural impulses which will eventually reach the various muscles of the articulators. The generated impulses descend via projection fibers that collectively form a group known as the cortico-bulbar tract. The impulses are somewhat modified and refined via interconnections with other cellular masses (nuclei) and via tract connections (synapses), at various levels, with incoming sensory information. As the tract enters the brain stem most of the fibers cross over to the opposite side (decussate) and synapse with lower motor neurons. These lower motor nuclei in the brain stem "relay" impulses along the peripheral nerves (cranial nerves) that provide innervation for the muscles of the head, neck, and face. Specific lower motor neurons have the responsibility of relaying impulses along specific cranial nerves. In turn, each of the efferent cranial nerves synapse with a given muscle or muscle group. Thus, innervation and movement of the articulators (vocal folds, soft palate, tongue, mandible, lips) may occur in a partially or completely simultaneous manner.

It is obvious that each articulator has the potential to move in a relatively independent manner. However, it is also true that their actions must be temporally coordinated in order to produce a desired affect. This requires that the neural commands for each articulator be formulated and specified in a partially or completely simultaneous, overlapping manner. Cooper (1966) refers to this as *parallel processing.* It seems clear that if different articulators are to move simultaneously, the neuromotor commands which underlie the physiology could not be specified in serial order but, rather, must be formulated and processed in a parallel manner. Cooper's concept of parallel processing has been widely accepted.

We have learned, as previously discussed, that we do not produce individual speech sounds as autonomous units. As has been pointed out, the individual articulator trajectories and targets will vary for a given phoneme depending upon such factors as phonetic context, rate of speech, and differential stress. The fact of coarticulation and the knowledge that the pattern of articulator muscle movements vary according to context tends to cast doubt on the candidacy of the phoneme as the neuromotor input unit for the production of speech. As Kozhevnikov and Chistovich (1965) suggest, the fact that we produce allophones and that speech is highly coarticulated suggests that the unit of speech must be larger than the individual phoneme. They suggest that our motor memory for speech would have to be unrealistically large if we were to store the neuromotor patterns for every allophone of every phoneme under all conditions of stress and rate of speech.

This hardly seems plausible. Even if our storage capacity were of sufficient magnitude to store the hundreds of thousands, possibly millions, of neuromotor patterns that would correspond to all the allophones, it is doubtful that expressive speech would develop as rapidly as it does in the child. Undoubtedly, if this were the case, articulation learning would extend well into adulthood.

This type of reasoning led Kozhevnikov and Chistovich to

suggest that the input units are probably syllable in size. Based on experimental observations of coarticulation affects, they suggest that "CV articulatory syllables" are the premotor input units. The model supposes that any number of consonants may precede the vowel and that while individual phonemes may be specified (commands generated) they are subordinate to the syllable as a whole. The model also proposes that the premotor commands are specified for the entire syllable with the first consonant. The implication is that left to right and right to left coarticulation affects may be accounted for by the fact that the individual phoneme commands are subordinate to, and are modified as a result of, the CnV articulatory trajectories and targets as a whole unit. Support from a number of studies is available. MacNeilage and DeClerk (1969), in a combined cinefluorographic and myographic study, examined coarticulation effects in a number of CVC syllables. They suggest that their results were consistent with a CnV sized input unit.

Some of the early investigations suggest that coarticulation effects result from the rather straightforward mechanical-timing limitations of the speech mechanism. The hypothesis is that since the onset and offset of articulator movements are not instantaneous there is some overlap among neighboring gestures. Thus, the targets for each phoneme, as specified pre-motorically, may not be completely achieved (articulatory undershoot) because of the mechanico-inertial and timing limitations of the speech mechanism. The position contends that once set into motion the articulators cannot stop abruptly and that this results in backward, left to right coarticulation. Right to left coarticulation affects are a bit more difficult to explain using this model.

However, Lindblom (1963), in studying vowel target undershoot under various conditions of syllable stress, suggests that an articulator moving toward a premotor command target may fall short of a target when it receives new instructions concerning the upcoming target(s). The articulator begins its movement toward the new target before it is able to complete the movement for the first target. Thus, anticipatory coarticulation is explained on the basis of a time-movement smear or blend among neighboring targets. Lindblom's target undershoot model suggests that the input units are phoneme in size and that coarticulation can be explained on the basis of natively sluggish articulators.

While appealing in its simplicity, the model hardly seems tenable in light of more recent research findings. For instance, it has been demonstrated in myographic research that different muscles come into play during the production of the same phoneme in different contexts (Harris, 1973). These data, combined with the observation that anticipatory coarticulation may span many consonants, tend to eliminate Lindblom's model from serious consideration. That is, although backward coarticulation may be explained on the basis of mechanico-inertial limitations of the mechanism, the model does not appear to be able to account for observed anticipatory coarticulation affects.

Along a somewhat similar vein, Oehman (1967) proposes a model that suggests that underlying articulation programming is a vowel to vowel diphthongal gesture. Oehman contends that articulatory vocal tract shapes for vowels are the primary target values in the program and that the amount of consonant coarticulation is simply a by-product of the degree of compatibility between the consonants' articulatory targets and the vocal tract shapes occurring between the two vowels. Although not clearly specified, it is assumed that the consonants would be independently generated and superimposed on the vowel to vowel gesture. Again, this model is not consistent with current research findings. In research where subjects produce a number of intervocalic consonants, the consonants differ in production not only as a result of the vowel contexts but also according to the neighboring consonants.

From the above we would certainly begin to think that Kozhevnikov and Chistovich's CV syllable model has merit. However, although not eliminating the syllable as a candidate for the basic input unit of speech, Sussman, MacNeilage, and Hanson did a study in 1973 that seriously challenges the "CV articulatory syllable" hypothesis. Studying subjects' productions of VCV syllables, they observed coarticulation effects from the first to the second vowel, spanning the consonant. Coarticulation effects spanning the medial consonant would certainly question the validity of the proposed consonant-vowel model. Further, the concept of individually programmed syllable-sized units return us to the question of learning, memory, and storage limitations. While fewer in number than all possible allophones, there is still an extremely large number of syllables that, accordingly, would have to be learned and stored.

One way out of this apparent contradiction to the syllable-sized hypotheses would be to accept Kozhevnikov and Chistovich's concept of higher level (CNS) reorganization. Although somewhat unclear from their model, we might assume that the individual phonemes and their corresponding neural commands undergo a cortical level reorganization (modification process) according to the overall shape and constituent target values of the syllables in which they are housed. Once reorganized, the syllable unit might be specified in a series of commands that overlap one another in time and are then fed forward to the neuromotor system in wholistic form.

Another model, not entirely disparate with the above, is proposed by Henke (1967). In Henke's model, the input units are phoneme in size, but the neural commands generated are composite bundles of "ideal" articulatory targets or goals. These ideal target values are based on a finite set of characteristics associated with each phoneme. Henke's model suggests that the stored units are these subphonemic articulatory characteristics and their associated articulator targets or goals. Since these are ideal (absolute) characteristics and targets, they are limited in number and, thus, would not exceed the storage capacity or learning ability of the child. Backward coarticulation is said to occur as the result of the mechanico-inertial limitations of the speech mechanism, as suggested earlier by Lindblom. Forward or anticipatory coarticulation effects are proposed to be the result of a "look ahead" or scanning mechanism that previews upcoming phonemes and modifies the targets of the phoneme being produced (coded) so that they are compatible. Thus, Henke's model would not restrict coarticulation to syllable boundaries and has been supported by a number of research investigations (Daniloff and Moll, 1968; Sussman, MacNeilage, and Hanson, 1973; Amerman, Daniloff, and Moll, 1970). Although appealing from a number of points of view, the model's reliance on mechanical restrictions to account for backward coarticulation is an apparent weakness. As previously stated, coarticulation research findings suggest that, in cases of left to right coarticulation different musculature or varying amplitudes of a single muscle contraction, will vary according to context. This indicates a higher level (premotor command level) organizational function than simple mechanical timing constraints.

As should be rather obvious by now there are presently more questions than available answers. Currently, there is no single universally accepted theory of the motor control and programming of speech production. However, the research continues. An understanding of this rather complex process would be of great value to the clinical speech pathologist. For example, if we knew the size and nature of the input units we could adopt stimulus material and therapy presentation modes that would correspond to the client's natural system. Certainly this would be facilatory. Recent studies on coarticulation have already begun to provide us with clinically relevant information. McDonald's work lay the foundation for using our knowledge of coarticulation in diagnostic, prognostic, and therapeutic activities. This will be discussed further in subsequent chapters.

Joint electromyographic-cineradiographic studies of normal velar coarticulation provide us with useful information in understanding the varying degrees of hypernasality in the speech of cleft palate children (Lubker, 1968; Kent, Carney, and Severeid, 1974). A 1975 study by Gallagher and Shriner examines articulatory inconsistencies in normal children's productions of /s/ and /r/ and demonstrates that more errors occur when the two sounds precede vowels than when they precede consonants. Similarly, Hoffman, Schuckers, and Ratusnik (1977) demonstrate that certain phonetic contexts are more facilatory than others with respect to children's ability to correctly articulate the /r/ sound. These investigators suggest that additional research is needed in this area and that such information would prove to be of significant clinical relevance. The author wholeheartedly agrees.

DISTINCTIVE FEATURES AND THE CONCEPTUAL BASIS OF SPEECH

In the foregoing discussion our focus was on the articulomotor (phonetic) nature of speech. We will now turn our attention to the conceptual (phonemic) basis of articulation. However, it is important from the onset that the reader realize that the two are not autonomously separate aspects of speech. Rather, they are highly interrelated. The term phonemic is used to designate consideration of the conceptual-cognitive underpinnings of articulation while phonetic refers to the external realization of speech through articulomotor processes. Although the two are unquestionably interrelated, the relationship is not necessarily a monotonic one. As discussed in the preceding section, all phonetic variations or gestures are not phonemic. In the word "pub," the initial and final consonants are obviously different phonemes. However, aspiration as a phonetic variation (initial consonant is aspirated while the final one is not) is irrelevant to our perception of the two as different phonemes. If aspiration was phonemically relevant, then the initial and final consonants in the word "pup" would be recognized as two separate sounds (phonemes). This is not the case. In the first example, voicing is the distinctive phonetic variation that allows us to classify (recognize) the two consonants as different phonemes. Thus, voicing is phonemically distinctive while aspiration is not.

Although there are a number of theories concerning the basic units of speech, it is widely recognized that the phoneme is one of the primary building blocks. There are approximately forty-five phonemes in the English language. Through them we are able to form words and express relationships (phono-morphemics). This process of using and combining phonemes to form units of meaning (semantic reference) is orderly and rule governed. The study of the process is called *phonology*. As a child we must learn the phonological rules if we are to communicate with others. For instance, certain phonemes may begin a word while others may not. The phoneme /ŋ/ may occur in the final position of a word but not in the initial position. Certain phonemes may be combined while other combinations are not permissible, e.g. /sk/ is a permissible combination while /zk/ is not. Thus, in addition to learning the phonemes of our language the child must also acquire the rules governing their correct usage.

Under normal conditions the average adult listener does not have any difficulty in recognizing and differentiating among the phonemes of our language. This is so because each phoneme has characteristics that allows it to be distinguished from each of the other phonemes. By analogy we might consider a child who is able to differentially name objects around him. He is able to do so because each object has intrinsic stimulus dimensions that distinguish it from other objects. Thus, when a child sees an object that is round, smells and feels like rubber, and bounces when you drop it, he labels it "ball." The stimulus dimensions matched his concept of "ballness." Further, he is able to differentiate it from the block next to it because the stimulus dimensions are distinctively different, e.g. the block is a three dimensional square, does not feel or smell like rubber, and does not bounce when you drop it. The child is able to recognize and differentially name the objects despite the fact that they have certain features in common (shared features), e.g. they are both small, can be held in the hand, and are play things.

The analogy breaks down, however, when you consider that unlike the practically endless number of stimulus dimensions (features) that allow us to differentiate among objects in our environment, the distinctive features underlying phoneme recognition are finite and relatively small in number. Just as words are formed by combining, in various ways, the forty-five phonemes of our language, phonemes are comprised of "bundles of distinctive features." While there are only a small number of features, combining them according to certain rules will allow us to form all of the phonemes of the English language.

It is apparent that some phonemes are more alike than others. This is so because they have more features in common and fewer feature differences than more dissimilar phonemes. The phonemes /p/ and /b/ are very much alike because they share all features except that of voicing. These kinds of phonemes are referred to as *minimal feature pairs* because they differ by only a single distinctive feature. While all phonemes have some feature(s) in common, they may differ by many. Phonemes that have more features in common with each other than they have feature differences are said to form a "natural phonemic class," i.e. plosives, fricatives, affricates, vowels, etc. The difference between any two phonemes may be determined by specifying their feature differences just as their similarity may be determined by specifying the feature attributes they have in common (shared features).

With the exception of place of articulation, distinctive features are binary, that is, have plus or minus attributes (the feature is either present or absent in the phoneme). For example a phoneme may be voiced or unvoiced, nasal or nonnasal. From this perspective distinctive features are contrastive and the change in a single feature attribute will result in a different phoneme. As an example, one of the feature attributes in the feature bundle comprising the phoneme /s/ is minus voicing. If this were changed to plus voicing the phoneme would become /z/. Likewise, if we were using a system that contained the feature *stop* and the attribute minus stop for the /s/ were changed to plus stop, the new phoneme would be /t/. Therefore, we might suggest that those phonetic variations (features) that signal phonemic change are contrastive and, thus, distinctive features. Distinctive features are an integral part of the phonemic conceptual system underlying speech articulation.

Singh (1976) defined distinctive features as "the physical (articulatory or acoustic) and psychological (perceptual) realities of the phoneme." This covers a great deal of territory, and it is not surprising that a number of very different feature systems have been developed. Some have assumed an articulatory reference with features designated in terms of voicing, place, and manner of articulation. Other systems have been developed with a predominantly acoustic or perceptual form of reference. Typically, separate systems have been developed for describing consonants and vowels. This has been necessary because of the total lack of commonality between the two along physiological, acoustic, and perceptual lines. Vowels are produced with a rather open, relatively static, vocal tract while consonant production involves highly ballistic movements of the articulators and requires close stricture or momentary closure of the tract. Vowels are periodic while consonants are aperiodic, or, in the case of voiced consonants, quasi-periodic at best. In other words, the feature systems for vowels would not relate to the feature specifications for consonants. From both a theoretical and clinical application perspective, this has generally not presented a problem. Articulation errors seldom occur across consonant-vowel boundaries, i.e. we seldom see a vowel for consonant or consonant for vowel substitution error. Since most articulation disorders involve consonants, we shall focus our attention on the consonant feature systems.

In order to be of clinical utility or even adequate from a theoretical point of view, a feature system must contain an adequate number of features to allow description of all consonant phonemes and to allow each phoneme to be differentiated from all others. As indicated above, each phoneme consists of a bundle of distinctive features, or more accurately, a bundle of attributes of the features in a given system. These may be visualized by listing the attributes under each phoneme in a feature *matrix*. Such a matrix also allows for easy visualization of phoneme contrasts according to feature attribute differences. As an example, Table I shows a feature matrix for a hypothetical language having only the six consonant phonemes p, b, t, d, k, and g.

For this language a two feature system is adequate. The binary feature of voicing (1 indicating the presence of voicing and 0 indicating its absence) and the trinary feature of place (1 indicating bilabial place, 2 indicating linguaalveolar place, and 3 indicating linguavelar place) are sufficient to identify the phonemes in a differential fashion. As can be seen, each phoneme differs from each other by at least one feature with a maximum difference of three distinctive features. The p-g and b-k pairs differ in voicing attributes and by two place attributes and are, therefore, maximally contrastive in the hypothetical, somewhat impoverished, language. It should be noted that our hypothetical language does not contain the feature *stop*. It is obvious that such a feature would be noncontrastive since there are no phonemes that would have a minus stop attribute and, therefore, such a feature would be irrelevant. By analogy, if the

TABLE I

FEATURE MATRIX FOR HYPOTHETICAL LANGUAGE
HAVING ONLY SIX PHONEMES

	p	*b*	*t*	*d*	*k*	*g*
Voicing	0	1	0	1	0	1
Place	1	1	2	2	3	3

entire world was blue without exception, the concept of color and "blueness" would be irrelevant and would probably not develop. It would appear that contrastiveness is extremely important to conceptual growth and development. This will be discussed further in Chapter 3.

One of the first distinctive feature systems to be developed was published by Jakobson, Fant, and Halle in 1952. Using spectrographic analysis of phoneme pairs, they initially identified twelve acoustically based features that they felt could be used to describe the phonological systems of languages universally. In fact, their purpose was to design a universally applicable system. All languages did not require all features. Thus, for English, only nine binary features were required to differentially define twenty-three consonants and six vowels: (1) Vocalic/Nonvocalic; (2) Consonantal/Nonconsonantal; (3) Compact/Diffuse; (4) Grave/Acute; (5) Flat/Plain; (6) Nasal/Oral; (7) Tense/Lax; (8) Interrupted/Continuant; and, (9) Strident/Mellow. Their feature matrix employed a plus-minus system, with "+" indicating the presence of the first feature element of each pair and a "−" indicating the presence of the second contrastive element. A complete description of each of the features may be found in the original publication or the interested reader may find summaries in books by Winitz (1969) and Singh (1976). The Jakobson, Fant, and Halle System, as Fant (1962) suggests, is limited in that it was designed more for the benefit of linguistic theory than clinical application.

In 1955, Miller and Nicely developed a system capable of distinguishing among sixteen consonants. They examined perceptual confusions among the consonants under various conditions of noise and filtering. In analyzing the confusions, they found five features that appeared to be maintained, i.e. the perceptual errors had the same features as the target. The five features were voicing, duration, affrication, place, and nasality. As is evident, even though the System is a perceptually based one, the authors used articulatory reference terms. For the four binary features, Miller and Nicely used a designation of one (1) to indicate the presence of the feature and zero (0) to designate its absence in a given consonant. The place feature is trinary with "0" designating front-of-mouth production in the consonants p, b, f, v, and m, "1" indicating midmouth place of production for the consonants t, d, θ, ð, s, z, and n, and "2" designating back-of-mouth constriction or closure for the consonants ʃ, 3, k, and g. While at first glance the Miller and Nicely System might be attractive to speech pathologists in light of the apparent simplicity, small number of features, and familiarity of terms, the System would not be highly useful from two points of view. First, the System is only able to differentiate among sixteen consonants. There are twenty-five in English. For instance the /r/ and /l/ phonemes are not included in the System and yet are two of the most frequently misarticulated by children. Second, the feature of "duration" would appear to be of questionable validity relative to phoneme specification in English.

Modifications and expansions of Miller and Nicely's System have been offered by Wickelgren in 1966, Singh and Black in 1966, and Singh in 1968 (Singh, 1976). Singh's 1968 System consists of eight features capable of differentially defining all twenty-five English consonants. Like the Miller and Nicely System, the reference is primarily articulatory and, with the exception of the place feature, uses a "0-1" bipolar designation frame. The features include voicing, nasality, frication, duration, liquid, glide, retroflex, and place. The "place" feature is quarternary with the four specifications: (1) to designate front or labial articulation, (2) midfront or alveolar production, (3) midback or palatal place of articulation, and (4) to designate back or velar articulations. The System would appear to have utility for the speech pathologist in analyzing articulation error patterns. However, we must await research validation on the "psychological reality" of all the features in the System before determining its absolute usefulness as a clinical tool.

Perhaps the most elaborate of the feature systems developed to date was proposed by Chomsky and Halle in 1968. In their System, phonological features purportedly specify the phonetic configuration and nature of the vocal tract. Since these phonological features specify phonetic "reality" and since all people, regardless of their native language, have similar vocal tracts, the authors view the System as having universal linguistic applicability. There are thirteen features in the Chomsky and Halle System: (1) vocalic; (2) consonantal; (3) high; (4) back; (5)

low; (6) anterior; (7) coronal; (8) round; (9) tense; (10) voice; (11) continuant; (12) nasal; and, (13) strident. All thirteen features are binary and, according to Chomsky and Halle, represent the *inputs* or abstract targets to be processed by the articulo-motor (phonetic) system. The process involves the generation of a set of appropriate phonological features (+ or − attributes of the thirteen above) for each phoneme to be produced. The attributes specify the configuration and nature of the vocal tract needed to produce the desired phoneme. If a single feature attribute is generated in error, the phoneme will be in error. The System is a complex one with the thirteen features defined as falling into one of five classes or feature types: Major Class Feature; Cavity Feature; Manner of Articulation Feature; Source Feature; and, Prosodic Feature. It should be mentioned that only eleven of the thirteen features are required to specify the English consonants. However, since articulation errors may consist of nonstandard English phoneme substitutions (distortion errors), the additional two are mentioned. The features *high, back, low, round,* and *tense* were included primarily to identify and differentiate among the vowels. The System has been criticized by a number of researchers on the grounds that many of the features do not appear to have psychological reality.

Recent techniques using multidimensional perceptual scaling procedures to discern psychologically real features would appear to offer promise. Systems designed by Singh, Woods, and Becker (1972) and Danhauer and Singh (1975) are examples. However, to date the procedures have not yielded a system capable of differentiating among all of the consonant phonemes of English. For this reason they would, as yet, be of limited clinical utility and will not be discussed here.

Distinctive feature systems and their clinical utility have been challenged by a number of researcher-clinicians. Leonard (1973) and Walsh (1974) suggest that most feature systems are too abstract and far removed from the physiological reality of speech production to be of clinical usefulness. Walsh suggests that "there is a gap between physical speech and mentalistic units" and proposes an elaborate articulatory feature system that specifies the exact manner, place, and voicing characteristics of production in anatomical and physiological detail. Leonard suggests that, while most feature systems may be adequate for binary abstract classification, they are generally inadequate at the level of phonetic description. He points out that although features may be binary at the conceptual level, coarticulation affects result in varying degrees of plus or minus representation at the phonetic level. For instance, nonnasal phonemes may evidence varying degrees of nasality when abutting with nasal phonemes, just as voiceless consonants may be partially voiced in the presence of voiced phonemes. Thus, abstract categorization and phonetic reality are somewhat disparate.

Faircloth (1974) used the Chomsky and Halle System and her own phonetic system to analyze the defective articulation of a four-year-old boy. She reports that the Chomsky and Halle System revealed only one feature (+strident) that was never produced by the child while her phonetic approach revealed that affrication and palatal place were never produced correctly. Faircloth stresses the point that manner and place of articulation considerations are important in evaluation and therapy planning. Similarly, distinctive feature systems have been criticized for their lack of utility in describing nonstandard or aberrant articulation errors, e.g. lateralization of the airstream, pharyngeal fricatives, glottal stop substitutions, etc.

These and other related arguments have led a number of speech pathologists to discard distinctive feature theory and to use the more traditional phonetic analysis methods. A few have designed "phonetic feature matrices" to maintain the concept of distinctive feature theory and, at the same time, to resolve some of the challenges discussed above. Table II reflects a typical phonetic feature matrix (prepared by the author solely for the purpose of example) that uses traditional place, manner, and voice designation.

The above criticisms of distinctive feature systems, however, may not be completely appropriate. As discussed earlier, distinctive feature theory concerns the phonemic-phonological bases of speech. Features are concepts, not necessarily phonetic realities. Distinctive feature analysis is designed to assess the client's phonemic system, not his phonetic production capability. Such an analysis ideally reveals what the child knows about the sound system; what features have been acquired and under what

TABLE II

PHONETIC FEATURE MATRIX BASED ON TRADITIONAL PLACE, VOICE, AND MANNER DESIGNATIONS

	p	b	t	d	k	g	m	n	ŋ	tʃ	dʒ	f	v	s	z	ʃ	ʒ	θ	ð	w	r	l	j	h	ʍ
Voicing	−	+	−	+	−	+	+	+	+	−	+	−	+	−	+	−	+	−	+	+	+	+	+	−	−
Nasal	−	−	−	−	−	−	+	+	+	−	−	−	−	−	−	−	−	−	−	−	−	−	−	−	−
Plosive	+	+	+	+	+	+	−	−	−	−	−	−	−	−	−	−	−	−	−	−	−	−	−	−	−
Fricative	−	−	−	−	−	−	−	−	−	−	−	+	+	+	+	+	+	+	+	−	−	−	−	+	+
Affricate	−	−	−	−	−	−	−	−	−	+	+	−	−	−	−	−	−	−	−	−	−	−	−	−	−
Liquid	−	−	−	−	−	−	−	−	−	−	−	−	−	−	−	−	−	−	−	−	+	+	−	−	−
Glide	−	−	−	−	−	−	−	−	−	−	−	−	−	−	−	−	−	−	−	+	−	−	+	−	+
Labial	+	+	−	−	−	−	+	−	−	−	−	−	−	−	−	−	−	−	−	+	−	−	−	−	+
Labiodental	−	−	−	−	−	−	−	−	−	−	−	+	+	−	−	−	−	−	−	−	−	−	−	−	−
Linguadental	−	−	−	−	−	−	−	−	−	−	−	−	−	−	−	−	−	+	+	−	−	−	−	−	−
Alveolar	−	−	+	+	−	−	−	+	−	−	−	−	−	+	+	−	−	−	−	−	+	+	−	−	−
Palatal	−	−	−	−	−	−	−	−	−	+	+	−	−	−	−	+	+	−	−	−	−	−	+	−	−
Velar	−	−	−	−	+	+	−	−	+	−	−	−	−	−	−	−	−	−	−	+	−	−	−	−	−
Glottal	−	−	−	−	−	−	−	−	−	−	−	−	−	−	−	−	−	−	−	−	−	−	−	+	−

rules they are being used for the perception and production of speech.

Pollack and Rees (1972) suggest that a child's defective articulatory behavior may represent an "ideolect" that reflects his phonological system. This is supported in a study by McReynolds and Huston (1971). They examined ten children with severe articulation defects using distinctive features analysis. The target features of the phonemes tested were recorded. Each child's productions were then analyzed in terms of the feature attributes present and these were compared to the target feature bundle for each phoneme. They found that children are consistent in their feature errors across phonemes and that a single feature error frequently accounted for multiple phoneme errors. This led them to hypothesize that articulation errors may occur as the result of either the feature(s) not being present in the child's repertoire or inappropriate feature applications. In the second case, the feature is present in the child's speech but is not being combined with other features according to the phonemic rules of English. From this we can understand that a child's misarticulations do not simply reflect an immature phonological development but, rather, may represent a complex system of rules that the child is using to generate the basic building blocks of speech. This deviant rule system is what Pollack and Rees are referring to when they speak of a child's "ideolect."

Articulation disorders do not always reflect simple phonetic production problems but frequently represent inappropriately developed phonemic rules. Compton (1970) emphasizes the same point when he indicates that a child's misarticulations are systematic and predictable when viewed from the phonological rule system of the child. Pollack and Rees suggest that distinctive features, as conceptual realities, rightfully belong to the acoustic-perceptual system and, therefore, cannot be appropriately applied to the articulomotor, phonetic aspects of speech production. They suggest, and the author agrees, that articulation errors may be classified as one of two major types: (1) *Phonetic Errors*, which reflect problems in the articulomotor execution of speech and generally occur as sequelae to neurophysiological or orofacial, structural deficits; and, (2)

Phonemic Errors, which reflect a deviant phonological rule system. Thus, many of the criticisms that have been leveled at distinctive feature systems and their applicability may have arisen out of inappropriate attempts to apply a phonemic system to a predominantly phonetically based question or problem. For example, pharyngeal fricative and glottal stop substitution errors typically occur in clients with velopharyngeal insufficiency and are therefore phonetically based.

The same may be true for lateralization of the airstream in sibilant productions, nasalization of nonnasal consonants, off-target articulatory distortions in dysarthria, etc. The client manifesting such an error pattern may well possess an adequate (normal) phonemic system, i.e. may have acquired all of the features of the language and have knowledge of the rules governing their correct usage, but may not be able to demonstrate it phonetically due to structural or physiological limitations. Rather than adopting an "either-or" attitude, however, it should be obvious that both articulophonetic and phonemic (distinctive feature) systems of analysis are warranted with each having a related but somewhat separate focus. Many of the problems seem to have come about because of a desire on the part of some to apply one, unitary system in the analysis of both the child's knowledge of the sound system as well as his ability to produce its elements.

The "reality" of selected distinctive features has been demonstrated in a number of studies employing different experimental paradigms. It has been demonstrated that in languages that have common features, children acquire the features in the same relative order, thus establishing linguistic universality. For instance, Menyuk (1968) demonstrates that Japanese and American children acquire the features *nasal, grave, voicing, diffuse, continuant,* and *strident,* in the same relative order (listed in order of first to last feature to appear). She reports that the features of "+nasal" and "+voicing" were the easiest to perceive and produce by both groups of children and suggests that features that are maximally different, i.e. have decided on and off characteristics, are acquired first, probably because they are the easiest to discriminate. Features with less polarity, such as place of articulation, are acquired later in the child's development. This will be discussed further in Chapter 3. Tannahill and McReynolds (1972) indicate that consonant speech sound discrimination varies according to the number of distinctive feature differences between contrastive phonemes. Discrimination becomes easier with an increase in the number of feature differences. This suggests that listeners use features in a very real way to distinguish among phonemes. However, Tannahill and McReynolds also report that all features used in the discrimination paradigm do not have equal weight and that the most discriminable features were voicing and affrication. The apparent lack of feature equality (perceptually) has been reported by a number of researchers using different research designs (Singh, 1971; LaRiviere, et al., 1974; Graham and House, 1971; Ritterman and Freeman, 1974).

The reality and applicability of distinctive features have also been demonstrated in experimental therapy approaches. Although a detailed discussion of therapy will be reserved for Chapter 7, it seems appropriate here to mention a study by McReynolds and Bennett (1972). The study is concerned with distinctive feature generalization in articulation therapy. Three children were taught to identify a target (error) feature using a discrimination approach in which each child was presented repeated minimal feature pairs (the two phonemes contained plus or minus attributes of the feature). Once able to identify the presence or absence of the feature with a fair degree of accuracy, the children worked on imitating the feature (selected phoneme containing the plus attribute of the feature) in first the initial and then the final positions of nonsense syllables. Posttherapy feature analysis revealed that the errors decreased by 69 to 84 percent and that generalization had occurred to phonemes not used in the therapy program. This finding lends further support to the conceptual reality of distinctive features and points to their potential clinical utility with phonemic articulation disorders.

Other evidence to support the reality of distinctive features may be drawn from dichotic listening research (Studdert-Kennedy and Shankweiler, 1970; Day and Vigorita, 1972; Johnson, 1975; and, Johnson, Sommers, and Weidner, 1978). These studies, as well as numerous others, repeatedly demonstrate the influence of manner, place, and voicing features in obtained dichotic ear preferences (hemispheric laterality). Certain features appear to require processing by the left hemisphere to a greater extent than others.

Thus, while all of the essential contrasts (features) of our language have not been empirically demonstrated, it should be clear that the theoretical and clinical utility of distinctive features is just beginning to be tapped. A good deal of evidence from multiple sources convinces the author that many of the traditional place, manner, and voicing features are indeed real. The use of distinctive feature theory in the evaluation and treatment of phonemically based articulation disorders is only in its neonatal stage of development. Examples of their utility will be presented in subsequent chapters.

ACOUSTIC PHONETICS AND THE PERCEPTION OF SPEECH

Any discussion of the nature of articulation would be incomplete without reference to the topic of speech perception. However, no attempt will be made here to provide the reader with exhaustive coverage of the topic. Books by Sanders (1977) and Massaro (1975) provide excellent reference for readers interested in in-depth discussion. The material presented here will be restricted to basic concepts and topics of central concern to articulatory perception. The two preceding sections on coarticulation and distinctive features have direct bearing on the various theories of speech perception.

Let us begin by pointing out that the physical world around us and our perceptions of it are not one and the same thing. They are different. Our perceptions are distorted biased transformations of physical reality. This is the case because we are not able to perceive the physical universe directly. Our neurophysiological systems are not directly receptive to it. Physical stimuli (reflections of the real world) must be transformed into a form that can be processed by our perceptual systems. This is the primary role of our sensory end organs (eyes, ears, etc.). They provide an interface between the real world and our central nervous systems. As an example, sound is created when an object is set into motion.

The motion or movement pattern of the object results in a

corresponding series of compressions and rarefactions of the molecules in the surrounding media (air). Neighboring molecules are affected, compressing and expanding relative to their rest states and sound travels. The frequency of the sound is dependent upon the rate of movement of the object and the corresponding number of compressions and rarefactions over time. Intensity is contingent upon the magnitude or amplitude of the excursion (displacement) of the molecules from their resting state. However, this acoustic energy cannot be directly perceived. It must be transduced to a state that is compatible with our central nervous systems. To accomplish this the ear transduces the acoustic energy to mechanical, then to hydraulic, and, finally, to a neuro-electro-chemical signal pattern that can be processed by our neurological perceptual systems.

Since we do not perceive the acoustic signal directly but rather a transduced form of it, the question is, "What is it that we actually perceive?" We apparently transduce and code, or re-code, changes in static, constant states. These constant, relatively stable or fixed states, e.g. atmospheric pressure, provide the foreground or baseline. The changes or deviations from constant states are what we acknowledge as stimuli. In order to be meaningful, however, these changes must assume some kind of pattern, i.e. must be orderly in their occurrence. It therefore seems appropriate to conclude that we transduce, code, and perceive the relative patterns of stimulations from the physical world around us. In this light, speech perception may be viewed as a complex form of pattern perception.

Speech, in its physical acoustic state, is a complex pattern of intensity-frequency interaction over time. The ongoing speech wave contains multiple patterns (information cues) which occur simultaneously. The listener is apparently able to extract or identify the salient features of a speech segment because of the "cue" value of specific acoustic patterns. Further, he is apparently able to identify multiple features of a given speech segment in a simultaneous parallel manner. However, prior to discussing some of the acoustic cues used by the listener to identify selected features, we should briefly turn our attention to the articulators and production.

As most readers will recall from their introductory phonetics course, speech sound may be produced in one of three ways. During quiet respiration air is exhaled from the lungs, passing through the trachea, open glottis, laryngo, and oropharynx and exits via the nasal or oral cavity openings. If, however, the vocal folds are adducted, air pressure will build up subglottically until the pressure overcomes the resistance of the folds. The folds will then be blown apart in an upward and outward undulatory fashion. The folds will then return to the midline position via the recoil action of the stretched folds and will then be "sucked together" via the Bernoulli Effect. This cycle will repeat itself many times in one second depending upon the mass, length, and tension of the folds and the amount of subglottic air pressure buildup. When the folds are lengthened there is a corresponding decrease in critical fold mass and an increase in tension along the length of the folds. This results in a relative increase in frequency of vibration. Increasing subglottic air pressure and air flow will result in a relative increase in intensity. At any rate, as the folds open and close on the outgoing air stream, pulses or "puffs" of air are produced. This results in a quasi-periodic (recurring) sound known as the glottal tone or *voicing*.

The fundamental frequency of voiced sound in males averages approximately 125 Hz; in females 225 Hz; and in children approximately 300 Hz. Voiced sound is complex, not sinusoidal, thus, it is comprised of a fundamental frequency (lowest frequency of vibration) and harmonics (overtones or whole number multiples of the fundamental frequency). The voiced sound at the level of exiting the larynx would sound like little more than a buzz. However, it is modified substantially as it passes through the speaker's vocal tract. Depending upon the size, shape, coupling, and tension of the supralaryngeal tract, the voiced energy at certain frequencies will be amplified (reinforced, intensified) while energy at other frequencies may be absorbed or damped. This is the process of *resonance*.

The frequency regions that have been reinforced are called *formant frequencies* or resonance bars. Since each person's vocal tract is slightly different in size and shape, the formant frequencies will differ somewhat from speaker to speaker. This accounts for voice quality differences. However, even though there are differences in inherent vocal tract configurations among speakers, there is enough similarity in the basic speech mechanism so that modifications in the size, shape, and coupling of the tract for the production of a given speech sound will result in a relatively stable relationship among the formants (for a given speech sound) across speakers. This is a relative relationship and should not be interpreted to be frequency region specific. Although there may be as many as six resonant frequencies (formants), only the first two or three appear to be important to the perception of speech. All of the vowels and approximately 60 percent of the consonants are voiced.

A second sound source for speech is achieved through constriction of the vocal tract at various levels. When two articulators are brought close together so that they approximate but do not close off the tract completely, the outgoing air stream rushes through the small, slitlike opening. This results in air stream turbulence and a frictionalized, aperiodic, noiselike acoustic pattern. The fricative phonemes are produced in this manner.

A third sound source involves the momentary, complete closure of the vocal tract at various levels with a resultant buildup of air pressure. Rapid release of articulator contact results in an explosive release of the impounded air. The acoustic pattern is characterized by a brief gap of no energy, corresponding to the moment of tract closure and pressure buildup, followed by an abrupt, short duration energy spike that corresponds to the release of impounded air. This type of pattern is characteristic of the stop plosive phonemes.

These three basic sound sources may occur in various combinations and to varying degrees for a given phoneme. For example, the /z/ involves two sound sources: voicing and the frictionalized component produced as the air stream rushes through the linguaalveolar/dental constriction.

Liberman and his associates (see reference list) at Haskins Speech Research Laboratories in New Haven, Connecticut provide us with a good deal of information on the specific acoustic patterns (cues) that apparently enable listeners to extract or identify some of the important features of speech. It appears that the identification of *voicing* is contingent upon the presence of energy below 300 Hz and the timing of voice onset relative to the beginning of the consonant. For instance, it has been demonstrated with stop plosives that if voice onset occurs within thirty milliseconds following the plosive release it will be perceived as voiced. Voice onset after thirty milliseconds apparently cues a voiceless phoneme to the listener.

Identification of *place of articulation* is cued primarily by the nature of the first two formant transition patterns to and from neighboring vowels. Ohde and Sharf (1977) demonstrated the importance of "the temporal order relationship between the vocalic transition and steady state vowels in the perceptual process." It has been suggested that the second formant is especially critical to identification of place information. For instance, the place information for the syllables /ba/, /da/, and /ga/ is provided by the slope of the second formant as it moves to the steady state portion of the vowel. A spectrographic display for /ba/ will show a slightly rising second formant while the transition pattern for /da/ is slightly falling or level and the slope of the second formant for /ga/ is sharply falling.

Certain characteristic acoustic patterns also serve as *manner* cues. For example, fricatives are apparently identified by constriction cues (aperiodic, noiselike components in the acoustic signal). Duration of the noise, bandwidth, relative frequency locations of the energy, and intensity may signal specific fricative phonemes. Plosives are apparently cued by a rapid, abrupt energy spike preceded by an energy gap. Unlike the consonants, which are highly ballistic and are produced with marked modifications in vocal tract configurations, vowels are relatively stable and are produced with a relatively open vocal tract. Thus, vowels show (spectrographically) a more steady energy pattern, i.e. there is less change in the acoustic pattern over time than we see for consonants. The identification of specific vowels is related to the relative frequency locations and interrelationships among the first three formants, as well as, the relative duration and intensity of the acoustic energy.

It would appear that we are beginning to identify some of the acoustic correlates of the salient perceptual features used by the listener in speech recognition. However, a more complex question and certainly one that is more difficult to answer arises. How, by what process, are these acoustic patterns processed: what internal operations are involved in the pattern perception of speech? At the present time we are still at the theoretical, model-building stage in our knowledge. However, research efforts have given us insights into the question and, as Sanders (1977) suggests, any model of speech perception must take into account what we already know about the process. Thus, our present knowledge provides us with some constraints on our theoretic meanderings and, at least, gives us some information on the possible shapes that a viable model would have to assume. There are several points that seem important, and these will be presented before discussing the models of speech perception per se.

First, it has been repeatedly demonstrated, through a number of experimental paradigms, that speech is processed differently than nonspeech stimuli. Speech is special and involves different neurological mechanisms than nonspeech auditory stimuli. Speech is perceived or discriminated *categorically*, i.e. our ability to discriminate between speech sound differences is only as good as our ability to identify (recognize and categorize) the two sounds. Acoustic variations within category (nonphonemic variations) are not discriminated. Nonspeech auditory stimuli are perceived continuously. For example, if we systematically increase the frequency of a pure tone a listener will be able to continuously perceive and discriminate among the various frequency levels of the tone. The same is not true for speech sounds. For instance, if we were to systematically modify the second formant transition pattern of /b/ until it became the same as that for /d/, the average listener would not discriminate among the changes until it achieved some critical level, at which time it would be perceived and coded as /d/. The speech mode is, therefore, said to be categorical.

Related to this first point is the fact that listeners are able to perceptually identify a given speech sound even though the acoustic signal is highly variable. We recognize the phoneme /d/ whether it is spoken by a child or an adult. Obviously the frequency information would be quite different. We also recognize the phoneme regardless of the phonetic context in which it is produced. This is also true for conditions of variable stress and rate of speech. As discussed in the first section of the chapter, coarticulation effects are readily demonstrable in the acoustic pattern. The /d/ in the syllable /di/ is acoustically quite different from the /d/ in the syllable /du/. However, we identify both of them as the same and recognize them as the phoneme /d/. This is referred to as *perceptual invariance* or constancy in the face of marked acoustic variance. This fact has proven to be a major stumbling block for a number of the older theories of speech perception. It is obvious that there cannot be a one to one absolute relationship between perception and the acoustic waveform. The waveform is different for each of the thousands of different allophones produced, for different speakers and for different speaking conditions. It is apparent that although we produce allophones the listener perceives phonemes.

A number of theories have been advanced in an attempt to explain this apparent paradox. Some have suggested that we are able to "normalize" or standardize the speakers speech patterns by making reference to our own production systems and vocal tracts. This position posits that after listening to a speaker for a short time we are able to generate an internal hypothesis about what the speaker has produced by comparing the segments to our own system of phonologic-phonetic rules.

Recent research suggests that perception is highly relative. For example, in a recent study by Miller (1977), it was demonstrated that the recognition of individual features is contingent upon the presence of other features in the speech segment. This position suggests that feature perception is not an independent absolute process but rather occurs as a result of the listener's analysis of the interrelated feature pattern in the variable acoustic waveform.

In addition to the categorical nature of speech perception and perceptual invariance in the face of acoustic variation, speech perception models must also be able to account for the findings concerning infant speech perception. Research using high amplitude sucking and heart rate dishabituation paradigms have pretty convincingly demonstrated that one- to three-month-old infants are able to discriminate between (although not necessarily in a meaningful way) differences in voicing and place of articulation (Eimas, 1974, 1975; Morse, 1974). These data suggest that the ability to discriminate between some of the salient, distinctive features of speech on the basis of acoustic characteristics is somewhat innate and that at least their non-meaningful distinction does not require learning. This has led a number of researchers to theorize the existence of innate, neurophysiologically based, linguistic feature detectors (Abbs and Sussman, 1971; Eimas, 1973).

In addition to taking the above into consideration, it would seem that any viable model of speech perception would also have to include a mechanism for the initial segmentation of the acoustic pattern in somewhat of a parallel manner. It would also have to incorporate a memory store for holding the salient segments while additional segments are being processed. Some mechanism for synthesizing or blending the individually processed segments into larger units of linguistic reference would also have to be postulated.

In the past there has been a good deal of discussion concerning the degree to which learning, language development and experience influence speech perception. On one side of the coin there have been those who have argued that perception is an *active* process, requiring learning and an ability on the part of the listener to, in some way, recode the speech signal. The counter argument has been that speech perception is a rather automatic process and that the listener possesses innate, species specific, speech detectors that enable him to recognize the salient characteristics of the acoustic waveform without any significant recoding or mediation. This has been referred to as the *passive* view.

In recent years we have come to recognize that neither position is completely accurate nor completely in error. Rather, it would appear that the early arguments were at least partially the result of viewing the process from different levels. It is reasonable to assume that both active and passive processes are involved. The early passive models generally proposed that via some type of template matching device or neurological filtering system, the listener is able to match or recognize the speech segment directly. These models assume a direct correlation between the acoustic pattern and recognition.

However, such models have largely been discarded since by themselves they are unable to explain the phenomenon of perceptual invariance in the face of substantial acoustic variation.

That is to say, if the acoustic information (waveform) is highly variable from speaker to speaker and from phonetic context to context, then how could we use a simple matching or filtering device? Likewise, however, those models that assume an entirely active process requiring learning and experience by the listener are unable to account for the research findings on infant perception. If the infant is able to detect differences in such features as voicing and place of articulation without first going through a reasonable period of phonological learning, then how can we assume a "recoding by rule," entirely active process? Thus, most of the contemporary models have attempted to incorporate both passive and active mechanisms, although they place varying degrees of emphasis on a certain "level" of the process.

Feature Detection Models suggest that the listener possesses receptive neural fields (certain patterns of neuron assemblies) that are selectively sensitive to certain patterns of stimulation. The position suggests that, although the acoustic signal is variable, a relative pattern will be representative of a specific speech segment and will trigger the receptive field. An example of such a model was proposed by Abbs and Sussman in 1971. Although these models have been classified as passive, careful inspection suggests active components. For instance, the Abbs and Sussman Model suggests that the receptive fields can be "selectively tuned" via a process of neural lateral inhibition of adjacent fields. This heightening of sensitivity of the field has long been posited to be one of the neural mechanisms underlying attention. This process unquestionably requires higher level, cortical involvement. Past experience with the language and linguistic sophistication undoubtedly are involved in the process in an "active" way. This writer has little doubt that such mechanisms are operative in speech perception, at least in the early stages of signal segmentation and detection. Meaningful recognition and synthesis, however, must require additional processing of this information.

As suggested earlier, speech appears to be processed differently, in a different mode and by different mechanisms, than nonspeech acoustic stimuli. A good deal of research evidence bears testimony to this point: the demonstrated categorical nature of speech perception; the fact that speech can be processed more rapidly than nonspeech; and, the results of EEG and dichotic listening research that demonstrate that speech is processed primarily by the left side of the brain, while nonspeech is processed, apparently equally well, by both hemispheres. These types of data have led a number of individuals to suggest that speech perception is intimately related to the process of speech production. It has been suggested that the perception of speech follows the same processing sequence as production only in reverse order. These theories have come to be known as *motor theories* of speech perception (Liberman et al., 1967).

Basically, the theories contend that the acoustic signal must undergo an auditory to phonetic transduction before recognition is possible. It is suggested that since the listener possesses knowledge of his own vocal tract, phonologic rules of production, and an auditory image of his own speech, he is able to recode and recognize what the speaker has said by running the machinery in reverse and generating the "abstract" neuromotor commands that would be necessary to produce a similar auditory pattern. This also explains the concept of "normalization" of the variant acoustic signals discussed earlier.

Proponents point to disturbances under delayed auditory feedback as additional evidence to support the theory and reciprocal relationship between production and perception. The motor theory has received wide-based support. However, it would suggest that some phonetic learning would be necessary. The infant research tends to challenge this position. We might also point to those children who do not acquire articulation skills but, nevertheless, seem to perceive speech and develop fairly good receptive language skills. It can also be pointed out that most research suggests that perception and comprehension precede production in development. This type of reasoning led Palmero (1975) to conclude that speech production is mediated by speech perceptual processes, the reverse of the motor theory. The issues are complex and, to date, the jury is still out. However, it is clear that perception and production are intimately related and, phylogenetically, evolved together in man.

A model that incorporates motor theory but proposes multiple levels of processing and is more specific in its detail is the *analysis-by-synthesis* model of perception (Stevens and Halle,

1967; Stevens and House, 1972). Basically, the model proposes that the acoustic signal first undergoes an auditory level analysis where it is transduced into temporal patterns and held in a memory store. Once sufficient pattern information is available to the system, phonetic features are extracted based on previously learned and stored patterns. When the phonetic information reaches the level of the syllable it is forwarded to a central speech analyzer mechanism. At this point, the listener supposedly generates an abstract phonetic hypothesis about the string and attempts to match it (the internally generated string) with the incoming signal. If a match occurs, the listener then generates the phonologic-phonetic rules governing production of the phonetic string and feeds these "articulatory instructions" to auditory memory where the corresponding auditory images are retrieved.

There are a number of variations on the theme but all suggest a repeated matching of the incoming signal with an internally generated set of articulatory gestures and with recognition occurring as the result of the synthesis of the matched units. These models would also seem to require some type of phonologic-phonetic learning as preliminary to perception and are not able to account for the infant perception findings.

A number of recent attempts have been made to combine the promising aspects of innate feature detectors with the mediational models (Eimas, 1974). It seems apparent that the neonate is able to detect differences in selected speech features. It is equally obvious that speech perception is a developmental process with meaningful organization and recognition requiring learning and relative mastery of phonological, syntactic, and semantic rules. Therefore, a viable model would have to include both. It seems reasonable to assume that we are brought into the world with a phylogenetically prewired neurological organization capable of detecting salient stimulus patterns such as speech. The concept of innate receptive fields for phonetic feature detection and discrimination is logical. However, we must distinguish between detection on the one hand and meaningful recognition and synthesis on the other.

Based on the present state of the art, it is the author's belief that the newborn is able to discern recurrent patterns of phonetic events represented in the acoustic waveforms of the speakers around him via innate feature detectors. With repeated exposure the child stores these patterns and becomes increasingly sensitive to their occurrence. He learns through repeated exposure that their occurrence is orderly and, in a progressive fashion, extracts (infers) the rules governing their occurrence. In this manner the child gradually develops a phonological store of the salient features and the rules governing their occurrence and combination possibilities. The young infant also demonstrates a progressively selective vocalization pattern that increasingly approximates the prosodic and segmental character of his speech models.

His early vocal play provides him with the opportunity to establish a motor memory or store of neuromotor commands and sequences needed to produce a given feature or feature pattern. Through repeated monitoring of his own auditory patterns and the tactile-kinesthetic-proprioceptive feedback information associated with selected neuromotor commands, he establishes a closed-loop system and a tie-in with the perceptual system. The size of the linguistic units that he is capable of processing and the corresponding complexity of their rules increases with linguistic experience and sophistication.

Semantic and syntactic development further delimit the phonological possibilities. During the early stages of phonological development the child's speech perception process is predominantly auditory, with incoming linguistic feature information combined and matched with stored information or patterns. However, as the child's production capabilities increase and phonological rule development becomes more complex, the child shifts his self-monitoring to greater reliance on tactile-kinesthetic-proprioceptive feedback information. This allows for greater speed and efficiency. As he does so he begins to mediate the linguistic feature information via his motor production rules. This allows the child to make more subtle discriminations than would be possible with a predominantly auditory analysis alone and perceptual sophistication increases. Although space does not allow a detailed consideration of the model, it suggests: (1) that children possess innate linguistic feature detectors based on neurophysiological receptive fields, (2) that through repeated exposure, children begin to detect-recognize feature patterns, infer the rules governing feature combinations and store the information, (3) that early speech perception probably involves a predominantly auditory type of internal matching of feature patterns, and, (4) that as the child develops a memory store of neuromotor commands and production rules and begins to monitor his own speech predominantly through tactile-kinesthetic-proprioceptive means, he begins to motorically mediate and recode the incoming feature information according to the principles of motor theory.

The relationship between the perception and production of speech is probably the most obvious in children with articulation defects. The high incidence of perceptual deficiency in the population has been well documented. While this will be discussed in subsequent chapters, a few additional points would seem to be warranted at this juncture. Traditionally, speech pathologists have viewed perception problems in terms of some kind of basic disturbance in auditory discrimination, memory, and/or sequencing. The question of course concerns the nature of such disturbances, i.e. what lies at the heart of such disturbances. In some children we can obviously point to basic disturbances in the mechanism.

From the above model, we might hypothesize that neurological disturbances could certainly disrupt the neurophysiological function of the receptive fields that are critical for feature detection. Such a disturbance would certainly result in deficiency in higher level functions, such as discrimination, synthesis, memory, etc. However, these children are probably in the minority. How do we account for perceptual deficits in children with apparently normal mechanisms? We must turn our attention to developmental issues.

The evidence to date suggests that the majority of the perceptual problems in articulatorily defective children arise from inadequate phonological feature and rule development, coupled with apparent deficiencies in the syntactic and semantic realms as well. Thus, the majority of the problems appear to reflect difficulty in the active mediation and recoding of the speech signal.

Recent support for this position was offered by Beasley et al.

(1974). They examined normal and articulatorily defective children's ability to assemble and produce segmented CVC syllables. Some of the syllables were meaningful (were mono-syllabic words) while others were nonmeaningful. They found that both groups of children had difficulty synthesizing the nonmeaningful syllables. However, there was a significant difference between the two groups in synthesizing the meaningful syllables. The children with articulation defects were significantly poorer at the task. Since there was no significant difference between the two groups on the nonmeaningful synthesis task but substantial difference when the task involved meaningful syllables, they conclude that the perceptual problems of the articulatorily defective children are probably not a reflection of a simple deficiency in auditory-speech waveform processing. Rather, they attribute the deficiencies to inadequately developed phonological-perceptual rule systems. They also suggested that stored semantic rules (constraints) probably play a significant role in the perceptual process. Support for this position can also be drawn from the fact that children with articulation defects have a higher than normal incidence of general language impairment and specific learning disabilities. These observations are meaningful and have obvious implications for the nature of perceptual training of articulatorily defective children in speech therapy.

REFERENCES

Abbs, J. and Sussman, H.: Neurophysiological feature detectors and speech perception. *J Speech Hear Res, 14:*23-36, 1971.

Amerman, J., Daniloff, R., and Moll, K.: Lip and jaw coarticulation for the phoneme /ae/. *J Speech Hear Res, 13:*147-161, 1970.

Beasley, D., Shriner, T., Manning, W., and Beasley, D.: Auditory assembly of cvc's by children with normal and defective articulation. *J Comm Dis, 7:*127-133, 1974.

Bloomfield, L.: *Language.* New York, HR&W, 1933.

Chomsky, N. and Halle, M.: *The Sound Pattern of English.* New York, Har-Row, 1968.

Compton, A.: Generative studies of children's phonological disorders. *J Speech Hear Disord, 35:*315-339, 1970.

Cooper, F.: Describing the speech process in motor command terms. *Haskins Laboratories Report on Speech Research,* SR-5/6, 1966.

The Nature of Articulation

Curtis, J.: The case for dynamic analyses in acoustic phonetics. *J Speech Hear Dis, 19:*2, 1954.

Danhauer, J. and Singh, S.: *Multidimensional Perception by the Hearing Impaired.* Baltimore, Univ Park 1975.

Daniloff, R. and Moll, K.: Coarticulation of liprounding. *J Speech Hear Res, 11:*707-721, 1968.

Day, R. and Vigorito, J.: A parallel between degree of encodedness and the ear advantage. *Haskins Laboratories Report on Speech Research,* SR-31/32:41-47, 1972.

DeLattre, T., Liberman, A., and Cooper, F.: Acoustic loci and transitional cues for consonants. *J Acoust Soc Amer, 27:*769-773, 1955.

Eimas, P.: Auditory and linguistic process of cues for place of articulation by infants. *Perception and Psychophysics, 16:*513-521, 1974.

————: Linguistic processing of speech by young infants. In Schiefelbush, R. and Lloyd, L. (Eds.): *Language Perspectives: Acquisition, Retardation and Intervention.* New York, Acad Pr, 1975.

Eimas, P., Cooper, W., and Corbit, J.: Some properties of linguistic feature detectors. *Perception and Psychophysics, 13:*247-252, 1973.

Faircloth, M.: Comparison of linguistic feature systems. *J Speech Hear Disord,* 376, 1974.

Fant, G.: Descriptive analysis of the acoustic aspects of speech. *Logos, 5:*3-17, 1962.

Gallagher, T. and Shriner, T.: Articulatory inconsistencies in the speech of normal children. *J Speech Hear Res, 18:*168-175, 1975.

Graham, L. and House, A.: Phonological oppositions in children: a perceptual study. *J Acoust Soc Amer, 49:*559-566, 1971.

Harris, K.: The physiological substrate of speaking. In Wolfe, W. and Goulding, D. (Eds.): *Articulation and Learning.* Springfield, Thomas, 1973.

Henke, W.: *Preliminaries to Speech Synthesis Based on an Articulatory Model.* Conference on Speech Communication and Processing. Bedford, Air Force Cambridge Research Laboratories, 1967.

Hoffman, P., Schuckers, G., and Ratusnik, D.: Contextual-coarticulation inconsistency of /r/ misarticulation. *J Speech Hear Res, 20:*631-643, 1977.

Jakobson, R., Fant, G., and Halle, M.: *Preliminaries to Speech Analysis.* Acoustic Laboratories, Massachusetts Institute of Technology, Tech. Report No. 13, 1952.

Johnson, J.: *The Clinical Relevance of Dichotic Ear Preference in Aphasia.* Doctoral dissertation, Kent State University, 1975.

————: In response to dichotic ear preference in aphasia: another view. *J Speech Hear Res, 21:*June, 1978.

Kent, R., Carney, P., and Severeid, L.: Velar movement and timing: evaluation of a model for binary control. *J Speech Hear Res,* 470-488, 1974.

Kozhevnikov, V. and Chistovich, L.: *Rech' Artikulyatsiya i Vospriyatiye,* 1965. Translated as Speech: Articulation and Perception. Washington, Joint Publications Research Service, 30, 543, 1966.

LaRiviere, C., Winitz, H., Reeds, J., and Herriman, E.: The conceptual reality of selected distinctive features. *J Speech Hear Res, 17:*122-133, 1974.

Leonard, L.: Some limitations in the clinical applications of distinctive features. *J Speech Hear Disord, 38:*141-143, 1973.

Liberman, A.: The grammars of speech and language. *Cognitive Psychol, 1:*301-323, 1970.

————: How abstract must a motor theory of speech be? *Haskins Laboratories Report on Speech Research,* SR-44, 1975.

Liberman, A., Cooper, F., Shankweiler, D., and Studdert-Kennedy, M.: Perception of the speech code. *Psychol Rev, 74:*431-461, 1967.

Liberman, A., Delattre, P., and Cooper, F.: Some cues for the distinction between voiced and voiceless stops in the initial position. *Lang Speech, 1:*153-157, 1958.

Liberman, P.: On the evolution of language: a unified view. *Cognition, 2:*59-94, 1973.

Lindblom, B.: Spectrographic study of vowel reduction. *J Acoust Soc Amer, 35:*1773-1781, 1963.

Lubker, J.: An electromyographic-cineradiographic investigation of velar function during normal speech production. *Cleft Palate J, 5:*1-18, 1968.

MacNeilage, P. and DeClerk, J.: On the motor control of coarticulation in CVC monosyllables. *J Acoust Soc Amer, 45:*1217-1233, 1969.

Massaro, D.: *Understanding Language.* New York, Acad Pr, 1975.

McDonald, E.: *Articulation Testing and Treatment: A Sensory-Motor Approach.* Pittsburgh, Stanwix, 1964.

McReynolds, L. and Bennett, S.: Distinctive feature generalization in articulation training. *J Speech Hear Dis, 37:*461-470, 1972.

McReynolds, L. and Huston, K.: A distinctive feature analysis of children's misarticulations. *J Speech Hear Dis, 36:*155-167, 1971.

Menyuk, P.: The role of distinctive features in a child's acquisition of phonology. *J Speech Hear Dis, 11:*138-146, 1968.

Miller, G. and Nicely, P.: An analysis of perceptual confusions among English consonants. *J Acoust Soc Amer, 27:*338-352, 1955.

Miller, J.: Non-independence of feature processing in initial consonants. *J Speech Hear Res, 20:*519-528, 1977.

Morse, P.: Infant speech perception: a preliminary model and review of the literature. In Schiefelbush, R. and Lloyd, L. (Eds.): *Language Perspectives: Acquisition, Retardation and Intervention.* Baltimore, Univ Park, 1974.

Oehman, S.: Numerical model of coarticulation. *J Acoust Soc Amer, 41:*310-320, 1967.

Ohde, R. and Sharf, D.: Order effect of acoustic segments of vc and cb syllables on stop and vowel identification. *J Speech Hear Res, 20:*543-554, 1977.

Palmero, D.: Developmental aspects of speech perception: problems for a motor theory. In Kavanaugh, J. and Cutting, J. (Eds.): *The Role of Speech in Language.* Cambridge, MIT Pr, 1975.

Pollack, E. and Rees, N.: Disorders of articulation: some clinical applications of distinctive feature theory. *J Speech Hear Disord, 37:*451, 1972.

Ritterman, S. and Freeman, N.: Distinctive phonetic features as relevant and irrelevant stimulus dimensions in speech sound discrimination learning. *J Speech Hear Res, 17:*417-425, 1974.

Sanders, D.: *Auditory Perception of Speech.* Englewood Cliffs, P-H, 1977.

Shankweiler, D., Strange, W., and Verbrugge, R.: Speech and the problem of perceptual constancy. *Haskins Laboratories Report on Speech Research,* SR-42/43, 1975.

Singh, S.: Perceptual similarities and minimal phonemic differences. *J Speech Hear Res, 14:*113-124, 1971.

———: *Distinctive Features: Theory and Validation.* Baltimore, Univ Park, 1976.

Singh, S., Woods, D., and Becker, G.: Perceptual structure of 22 prevocalic consonants. *J Acoust Soc Amer, 52:*1698-1713, 1972.

Spriestersbach, D. and Curtis, J.: Misarticulation and discrimination of speech sounds. *Q J Speech, 37:*483-491, 1951.

Stevens, K. and Halle, M.: Remarks on analysis by synthesis and distinctive features. In Wathen-Dunn, W. (Ed.): *Models for the Perception of Speech and Visual Form.* Cambridge, MIT Pr, 1967.

Stevens, K. and House, A.: Speech Perception. In Tobias, J. (Ed.), *Foundations of Modern Auditory Theory.* New York, Acad Pr, 1972.

Studdert-Kennedy, M. and Shankweiler, D.: Hemispheric specialization for speech perception. *J Acoust Soc Amer, 48:*579-594, 1970.

Sussman, H., MacNeilage, P., and Hanson, R.: Labial and mandibular dynamics during the production of bilabial consonants: preliminary observations. *J Speech Hear Res, 16:*397-420, 1973.

Tannahill, J. and McReynolds, L.: Consonant discrimination as a function of distinctive feature differences. *J Auditory Res, 12:*101-108, 1972.

Walsh, H.: On certain practical inadequacies of distinctive feature systems. *J Speech Hear Disord, 39:*32-43, 1974.

Winitz, H.: *Articulatory Acquisition and Behavior.* New York, Appleton-Century-Crofts. P-H., 1969.

CHAPTER 2

Important Variables in Articulation

SERVOSYSTEM THEORY

THE IMPORTANCE OF *feedback* to the acquisition and maintenance of human behaviors cannot be overstated. Although
many behaviors may be somewhat biologically predisposed, it is
only through the monitoring of our actions via our own sensorium and through the reactions of others that we are able to
refine, modify, establish, and maintain the behavior.

The child development literature in a variety of professional
disciplines supports the idea that behavioral development pro-
gresses from the gross, somewhat undifferentiated behaviors
seen in the newborn, to the fine, more sophisticated behaviors
manifest in adults. It would seem that there is a positive relationship between the complexity of a given behavior and the degree
of reliance on feedback. As a child develops behaviors that are
more complex, require finer motor skills and are more highly
differentiated, there is a somewhat proportional increase in the
amount of requisite feedback information. There seems to be
little question that the child must reach some level of
neurophysiological and structural readiness prior to being able
to meaningfully recognize and integrate feedback information
(Lenneberg, 1967).

However, biological readiness alone does not insure the
emergence of a behavior. This is certainly true for behaviors,
such as speech, that require complex fine motor control. In
addition to organismic readiness, certain minimum psycho-
social-environmental conditions must be present and the child
must be able to use and integrate multiple forms of feedback
information. Further, an individual's fine motor movement potential must be sufficient to support the complex, rapidly alternating movement sequences required for speech production.

44

In 1954, Fairbanks proposed a model of speech production that characterized the process as a *closed loop servosystem*. As differentiated from an open loop system, a closed loop mechanism requires feedback information concerning the nature of its output in order to operate smoothly or "as intended." Thus, Fairbanks' Model is comprised of *control, effector,* and *sensor* components. The control unit is undoubtedly a cortical level operation consisting of multiple levels of processing. It involves the processes of linguistic formulation and the subsequent recall of the motor movements, sequences, and targets needed to achieve given articulatory effects.

Fairbank's Model also supposes that the control unit possesses a comparator mechanism. The comparator receives information concerning the intended linguistic units and articulatory targets as they are generated. Neuromotor commands are generated and forwarded to the neuromotor (effector) system for execution. As the articulators are set into motion and the acoustic pattern is created, the multicomponent sensor mechanism comes into play. It registers such information as the speed, direction, and magnitude of articulator movement and the articulatory and acoustic targets achieved by the effector system. This information is transmitted to the comparator where comparisons are continually made between the intended targets and the achieved target values. If a match occurs, the speech process continues. If a disparity is noted, however, correction information is forwarded to the generator for modification purposes.

The exact neurophysiology underlying the process remains somewhat unclear. We do know, however, that there is not complete correspondence between the motor impulses leaving cortex and those arriving at the articulatory musculature. The neural transmission is modified and refined along the way in a manner consistent with given articulatory trajectory and target values. This is possible, in part, because we are able to sense (monitor) the movements that have been initiated and to make predictive decisions concerning needed adjustments via comparisons between intended output and realized probable output profiles (Hardcastle, 1976).

The sensor component probably underlying our ability to make "midcourse" corrections in movement is *proprioception*.

Proprioceptive feedback provides us with information concerning the position(s) of our articulators at a given point in time. It is made possible by sensory cells in the muscles (intrafusal fibers), joints, and tendons. The information is forwarded, via afferent tracts, to both cortex and cerebellum. For rather automatic or highly learned forms of behavior, it is believed that the cerebellum functions as a coordinating and proprioceptive monitoring center.

Tactile (touch) information is also shared by both cortex and cerebellum. Tactile information is made possible by more superficially located sensory nerve endings. The system provides information concerning the localization or point of contact between two articulators, the magnitude of the depression (force of contact) and time of contact and release. While proprioceptive and tactile information are both used in monitoring speech (taken together they are referred to as *kinesthesia*), it is doubtful that the latter would be very useful in midcourse correction activity because the movement would be over by the time such information had been analyzed.

The third component of the sensor system is *auditory* feedback. The end organ is the cochlea. The sensory receptors in the cochlea (hair cells in the Organ of Corti along the basilar membrane) respond to both air and bone conducted auditory signals. Information concerning frequency, intensity, and duration is projected to the thalamus via the eighth auditory nerve and from thalamus to the auditory cortex in the temporal lobe. Because it involves the transmission of sound through air and bone media, auditory feedback is slower than tactile or proprioceptive and arrives after the motor event has occurred. Like tactile feedback, however, it can provide information concerning the targets obtained and may provide the comparator with the types of confirmatory information needed to make *post hoc* corrections.

It seems clear that sensory feedback is vital to the closed loop system and that the development of articulatory skills, as well as the maintenance of articulatory accuracy, are dependent upon it. In extreme cases of sensory deprivation, such as congenital deafness, the failure to develop normal speech is at least partially attributable to the child's inability to monitor his vocalizations and speech attempts. As will be discussed later in the chapter, experimentally induced disruptions in either the auditory or kinesthetic feedback channels may result in disturbed or imprecise articulation.

The question of the weight or relative importance of the individual sensory channels to speech monitoring and control has been investigated by a number of researchers. For example, it has been suggested that vowel quality, pitch, and nasality are monitored primarily by the auditory channel while consonant production and accuracy may be monitored primarily via the tactile-proprioceptive feedback channels (Hardcastle, 1976; Ringel, 1970; Gammon et al., 1971). However, due to the complexity of the mechanisms involved and the apparent interactive, somewhat synergistic, nature of sensory feedback, such conclusions would seem to be premature.

Experimental attempts to induce sensory deprivation in a single channel are frequently confounded by the possibility of untoward contamination of other feedback channels. Further complications arise when one considers that the relative importance of a given sensory channel may well vary according to age and level of articulatory development. For instance, Van Riper (1958) suggests that early, during the child's learning and acquisition of the sound system, reliance on the auditory channel is primary. However, he suggests that as the child masters the required movement sequences for production he undergoes a shift in primary sensory monitoring with greater emphasis on the kinesthetic channels.

The hypothesis that the type of feedback important during the acquisition stage is different from that needed to control established behaviors is tenable and has been a recurrent theme in much of the literature in speech pathology. However, to the author's knowledge, the hypothesis has never been experimentally tested. Although the design problems are substantial, investigation in this area is badly needed and definitive information would possess a high degree of clinical and theoretical relevance.

It seems clear that the babbling and vocal play of the child during the first year of life represents more than a simple reflection of a contented baby. It provides the developing child an opportunity to establish correspondence between acoustic product, associated kinesthetic feedback, and the neuromotor commands required to produce specific vocal patterns. In other words, it affords the child the opportunity to begin establishing closed loop control.

During early infancy, vocalizations are general and nonspecific to the particular language of his parents. However, this early experience undoubtedly is of benefit in allowing the child to develop relatively gross motor control of the articulators and to record the acoustic and proprioceptive-tactile by-product of neuromotor execution. This would be analogous to the infant's early hand and finger play. While such movements may be partially random and nonskill or task specific, the behavior nonetheless allows the infant to begin development of manual dexterity and provides the opportunity for the establishment of kinesthetic and visual patterns (feedback) associated with such movements. This preliminary "play" is obviously vital to the child's later development of skilled, task-oriented visual motor (eye-hand) skills. Similarly, the infant's early vocal play is important to the later development of the skilled purposive movements needed for speech.

As the infant develops he begins to "compare" his own vocalizations (auditory) with those of his parents (this will be discussed further in Chapter 3). When the acoustic patterns are similar, the auditory image is highlighted and stored together with the corresponding oral sensory feedback and the neuromotor commands used to generate the movement sequences. This early need for *self-hearing* and auditory matching activity is undoubtedly the basis for the position that the auditory channel is primary during the acquisition stage of development. As discussed previously, once the child is comfortable with the "match" and once the auditory image has been subjectively stabilized, together with the oral sensory information, the child shifts primary monitoring responsibility to the kinesthetic channels. From this perspective, the auditory channel is primarily important in the initial establishment of the auditory image and for providing the comparator with correction information during the early phases of sound production learning.

The reader should not interpret the above as suggesting that once the child has obtained relative mastery of sound production they totally disregard auditory feedback information. It is only suggested that once the programming is relatively complete and speech comes under *internal* closed loop control the magnitude of the reliance on the auditory channel diminishes in favor of kinesthetic dominance. This has been the rationale underlying many hours of articulation therapy focused on reestablishing and heightening the child's auditory awareness and self-hearing ability. It has been suggested that the child must focus his auditory attention on the correct sound pattern, be able to hear his own error pattern and, through auditory comparisons, make the necessary corrections in his "program."

Although quite simplistic when compared to the neurophysiology underlying the processes, the servosystem model of speech production discussed above has provided a framework for conceptualizing articulation disorders. For example, we may envision deficiencies in the control unit in terms of either a deviant linguistic program (inadequate or deviant phonology) or problems in motor memory (recall and sequencing of appropriate targets and neuromotor commands). Problems with the effector unit may manifest themselves in imprecise articulation and occur secondary to neuromotor weakness or incoordination. Deficiencies in the multicomponent sensor unit may interfere with both the acquisition and maintenance of articulation skills. Of course the degree and particular type of articulation impairment manifest will be somewhat contingent upon the particular sensor mechanism involved (auditory, tactile, proprioceptive), whether the involvement is primarily sensory or perceptual or both and the magnitude of the disturbance.

While this may seem like a rather straightforward way of conceptualizing articulation disorders, it becomes complex and difficult to segmentalize when one realizes that control, effector, and sensor units function in an overlapping, interactive manner. The acquisition and establishment of the articulatory program both in terms of the linguistic (distinctive features and phonological rules) and motor memory elements requires adequate sensory feedback. Thus, a deficient control unit may reflect an underlying deficiency with the sensor unit.

The reciprocal may also be true. If one accepts an active model of speech perception, as discussed in Chapter 1, then apparent problems with the sensor unit in terms of auditory or kinesthetic discrimination may, in reality, reflect a deficiency in the recoding (mediation) of speech by an inadequately developed or defective control unit. Further, the closeness between the effector and sensor units is such that they are frequently referred to as a single sensorimotor system. As previously discussed, neuromotor impulses descending from cortex are modified by incoming sensory information. Thus, a deficiency in one system may adversely affect the other. This multiple interaction among systems makes a simple compartmentalization of articulation disorders almost impossible. However, regardless of the etiology or origin of the problem, the research literature has been quite stubborn in suggesting a relationship between articulation disorders and the presence of sensory and motor defects. Specifically, deficiencies in auditory discrimination, oral form discrimination and oral fine motor skills have been frequently cited.

AUDITORY DISCRIMINATION

Probably no other single variable has been given as much attention by speech pathologists as auditory discrimination. For the past forty years it has been suggested, with some variations on the theme, that underlying or occurring concomitantly with articulation disorders is a deficiency in auditory discrimination ability. This has provided the impetus for speech pathologists spending many hours with clients in auditory discrimination training, either preliminary to more direct methods of articulation therapy or concurrent with them. The relationship has been experimentally investigated using a wide variety of discrimination measures with both children and adults. Speech and nonspeech (pitch, loudness) auditory discrimination skills have been examined.

One of the first studies to compare normal and articulation impaired children was reported by Travis and Rasmus (1931). Using a 366 item speech sound discrimination test consisting of paired nonsense syllables, they examined normal and mildly articulation impaired children in the elementary school grades. They report that the articulation impaired youngsters performed more poorly on the discrimination task than their normal counterparts.

The findings of Travis and Rasmus gave rise to at least a dozen major investigations spanning a twenty to twenty-five year period *(see* Winitz, 1969 *for review)*. Some of these investigations report positive correlations between articulation defectiveness and auditory discrimination impairment while others failed to find such a relationship. In 1957, Powers reviewed the major reported findings and suggests a somewhat equivocal picture. She suggests that the weight of the evidence failed to support a systematic relationship. However, subsequent studies since that time, with the exception of studies by Prins (1962) and Shelton, Johnson, and Arndt (1977), overwhelmingly support the existance of a relationship.

In 1967, Weiner reviewed the literature and concludes that a positive relationship between articulation and auditory discrimination impairment "is almost invariably found in studies of children below nine years of age, and seldom found above that level." He offered this as a viable explanation for the rather disparate results reported in the early literature. Winitz (1969) also did an extensive review of the literature and supports Weiner's report.

In 1958, Wepman designed a test of speech sound discrimination that consists of forty word pairs. For thirty of the pairs there is a single phoneme difference while for the other ten pairs the words are identical. The task involves having clients make "same-different" judgments following the presentation of each pair. The child's error score is used to estimate an age equivalent with regard to developmental auditory discrimination ability. The test is mentioned here because it was widely adopted by practicing speech pathologists as a measure of discrimination ability. Although it remains in clinical use today, it has been challenged as a valid measure. However, using his test, Wepman (1959) investigates the relationships between obtained discrimination scores and articulation and reading impairment in elementary school aged children. He reports significant correlations and, based on his findings, hypothesizes that developmental delays in auditory discrimination are probably causally related to articulation and reading deficiencies.

Another factor that may be partially responsible for the inconsistent findings of the early research investigations, in addition to the age of subjects studied, is the severity of articulation impairment. A number of studies suggest that the relationships between impaired articulation and auditory discrimination ability is most reliably present in subjects with more severe articulation disorders (Cohen and Diehl, 1963; Farquhar, 1961; Sherman and Geith, 1967; Stitt and Huntington, 1969; Sommers, Meyer, and Furlong, 1969).

In the 1969 study by Sommers, Meyer, and Furlong, a large number of articulatory defective children in grades three through six were compared with a matched group of normal children using both pitch and speech sound discrimination measures. Of major importance was their finding that although the children with mild articulation defects performed similarly to the normal children, those subjects with severe articulation impairments demonstrated significantly inferior speech sound discrimination ability. In 1974, Sommers stated that "the weight of experimental evidence indicates that children with functional misarticulations are likely to have inferior speech sound discrimination." However, he qualifies his statement somewhat by indicating that while children with severe articulation impairments may have general problems in speech sound discrimination, those with only a few phonetic errors will probably have difficulty only in discriminating their particular error sounds.

Spriestersbach and Curtis (1951) report on a 1949 study by Anderson that demonstrates that children had greater difficulty in correctly discriminating the /s/ phoneme in contexts that result in their misarticulating the sound than in error free contexts. This connection between production and discrimination has subsequently been demonstrated by Aungst and Frick (1964) and Monin and Huntington (1974).

Aungst and Frick find that children with /r/ defects have more trouble in correctly identifying the /r/ sound in contexts in which they misarticulate the sound than in nonerror contexts. Of equal importance is their finding that discrimination ability is related to consistency of misarticulations only when the discrimination measure involves the child's comparing his own productions with those of an external model. They report that the results of traditional discrimination testing (Wepman's Auditory Discrimination Test) are not significantly related to their subjects' articulation performances. This has led to the suggestion that clinically relevant measures of auditory discrimination must include having clients judge the accuracy of their own productions with those of an external model.

In summary then it would appear: (1) that there is a high incidence of auditory discrimination impairment in children with articulation disorders, (2) that the relationship between auditory discrimination and articulation disorders is most obvious in children below nine years of age, (3) that children with severe articulation disorders (more than four phoneme errors) have generalized auditory discrimination impairments that may well manifest themselves on a traditional test of auditory discrimination ability, (4) that children with mild articulation disorders (only a few phoneme errors) may only have difficulty in correctly discriminating their own error sounds and, more specifically, in phonetic contexts which house the error sound; and (5) that the most clinically useful and relevant type of discrimination testing involves having clients judge the accuracy of their own productions with those of some external model.

As mentioned earlier, there would appear to be a fairly strong correlation between discrimination and production. This would offer support for the motor theory of speech perception discussed in Chapter 1. In 1968, Locke suggested that phonemic perception may well involve a process of motor mediation. He proposes that speech sounds which are acoustically very similar may be differentiated (discriminated) by coding them in terms of their articulomotor production and using the more distinctive information of muscle actions, articulatory movements and targets for making discriminative comparisons.

From this perspective, faulty discrimination might then be the result of an inability to mediate between two acoustically similar sounds on an articulomotor level. From this position it is easy to see why a child with articulation errors such as a /w/ for /r/ or /f/ for /θ/ substitution would manifest specific discrimination difficulty with his error sound. That is, since the error and target phonemes are acoustically similar and produced the same, the child would not be able to differentiate between them on an articulomotor level. As pointed out by Locke, it might also explain why place of articulation errors are frequently the most common type of error in the child's speech. Others suggest that the child may, in reality, be able to discriminate between his error sound and the target phoneme, but because he perceives them as allophonic variants of the same phoneme, does not acknowledge them as "different."

However, as distinct from the motor theory position, it has been suggested that correct perception and discrimination precede production. Many suggest, and perhaps the majority of speech pathologists agree, that the child first establishes a conceptual acoustic image of the phoneme and then, through trial and error, feedback, and reinforcement, attempts to match his articulatory output to it. Faulty discrimination is then usually attributed to some kind of basic disturbance in the child's ability to analyze and process the acoustic signal.

This has been the rationale for significant portions of therapy time being devoted to activities designed to enhance the child's ability to identify and hold sequential auditory events in memory and to discriminate among a variety of speech and nonspeech auditory stimuli. In fact, it has been demonstrated that auditory discrimination ability can be improved via a feedback and reinforcement paradigm (Berlin and Dill, 1967) as well as through simple vicarious learning (Ritterman, 1970). Additional support for this position may be drawn from the fact that a number of researchers report that articulatory defective children have difficulty not only with speech sound discrimination but with discrimination tasks involving pitch and loudness judgments as well (Stitt and Huntington, 1969; Sommers, Meyer, and Fenton, 1961; Mange, 1960).

It has also been demonstrated that there are relationships among impaired articulation, auditory discrimination, and language skills (Stitt and Huntington, 1969; Marquardt and Saxman, 1972; Perozzi and Kunze, 1971). It is quite possible that in young children defective auditory discrimination may be a source of covariance for both defective articulation and deficiency in selected language skills and may be causally related to both. However, at this point in time such a statement is highly speculative and the issue certainly warrants further investigation.

As suggested earlier, it may well be that early in the child's phonological acquisition period auditory discrimination is of paramount importance and highly influential with reference to the child's speech production abilities. Menyuk (1968) hypothesizes that children's ability to discriminate among sounds on the basis of distinctive feature differences is significant to their phonological development. She states that those features that have decided on and off characteristics are the easiest to discriminate and are, therefore, acquired first. She also indicates that children who are developing normally show only single feature differences in their sound production errors.

Similarly, Tannahill and McReynolds (1972) demonstrate that phonemes differing by many distinctive features are easier to discriminate than phonemes differing by only a single feature. It would appear that those sound pairs that differ by only a single distinctive feature and are difficult to resolve auditorily (such as subtle place of articulation differences) are differentiated later in the child's development. Discrimination of these types of pairs may well require the establishment of closed loop control and primary reliance on kinesthetic feedback and subsequent motor mediation as Locke suggests.

Although speculative, it may well be that there are at least two basic underpinnings for observable deficiencies in auditory discrimination. The first may involve a fundamental disturbance in the processing of the acoustic waveform with resultant deficiencies in the segmentation and identification of meaningful speech and nonspeech auditory stimuli, auditory memory, and discrimination. Such deficiencies might result from neurological disturbances involving the "receptive fields," as discussed in Chapter 1. Such disturbances could undoubtedly result in severe articulation disorders, as well as deficiencies in the acquisition and development of a number of language skills. However, as Beasley et al. (1974) suggest, "evidence to date supports the contention that articulatory disordered children are not simply deficient in their perceptions of the speech waveform, but that other factors are operating which contribute to articulation disorders" (p. 132). The authors were referring to the importance of phonological rules and semantic constraints in speech perception.

If one accepts that active processes are involved in speech

perception, at least at some level of processing, then some auditory discrimination deficits may spring from a deficient phonological system. That is, a problem in discriminating between two speech sounds may result from an underdeveloped or deviant phonological code that does not distinguish the two phonemes. In this case, we would expect to see rather specific discrimination problems involving speech only and, more specifically, the child's error sounds. In keeping with the research literature, this may be the case in the majority of "mild" articulation disorders where only a few sound misarticulations are present. Consideration of this matter is extremely important to clinical management and decision making concerning the amount and type of auditory discrimination training that may be needed by a given client.

It has been said that an intelligence test tests what the intelligence test tests. The degree to which we accept test scores as indicative of "intelligence" reflects the degree to which we accept the assumptions underlying test construction as valid. Such test scores may be shown to be highly predictive of clients' performances on other tests or specific tasks or accomplishments. However, even in this case we must assume that the "other tests" or tasks or accomplishments are, in some way, valid reflections of the variable in question, namely intelligence. The same can be said of tests of auditory discrimination ability. The problem would seem to revolve around the fact that there is no absolute external criterion with which to compare tests to determine if they are indeed valid indices of auditory discrimination ability.

Some research has been done in an attempt to delineate the performance characteristics of children on certain types of tests and attempts have been made to improve the face validity of tests based on our knowledge of the nature of speech. For instance, tests that involve having clients judge two competing sounds presented in isolation or even in word contexts are certainly not consistent with the "natural" type of discriminations a child makes as he listens to ongoing connected speech.

Schwartz and Goldman (1974) find that not only are stimulus contexts important, but that the presence or absence of background noise is an important variable. They suggest that testing speech discrimination ability in a quiet, sterile room is artificial and may be misleading. The point seems to be that children do not make discriminations in their natural environments by listening to individually spoken sounds or words under conditions of extreme quiet. Testing under these conditions may then lead to an unrepresentative sample of their ability under normal, day to day conditions. Similarly, having a client make binary categorical judgments, such as "same or different," may be artificial and impose a restriction that camouflages actual discrimination ability.

The nature of the competing sound pairs would also seem to be an important consideration. As previously discussed, Tannahill and McReynolds demonstrate that the ease of discriminating between two phonemes is related to the number and type of distinctive feature differences. It has also been shown that those sounds receiving primary stress and occurring in the final position of words are more easily discriminated correctly (Knaffle, 1973; Blasdell and Jensen, 1970). These and other considerations have all too often not been given adequate consideration in test construction. Measures of a client's ability to accurately compare and contrast his own articulations with those of others and, finally, to recognize his misarticulations as errors would appear to offer the highest degree of clinical validity. However, we are in need of additional research and a standardization of procedures that would allow clinicians to "speak the same language" when discussing auditory discrimination.

ORAL STEREOGNOSIS

The bulk of the experimental concern about a possible relationship between disturbed feedback and articulation disorders has centered on auditory discrimination. Certainly this is the case with the earlier literature and somewhat true today. However, in the literature of more recent vintage, beginning primarily in the 1960s, there has been an emergence of hypotheses concerning the possible relationship between articulation disorders and nonfunctional disturbances in oral sensory awareness and discrimination. A number of researcher-clinicians suggest such a relationship and speculate that if impaired oral sensory discrimination ability is not causally related to articulation disorders then it is, at least, a predisposing factor capable of attributing to such. Many have followed up on such reasoning by speculating that perhaps the majority of so-called "functional" articulation disorders are in reality attributable to organic deviations in oral sensory and/or motor ability. This is not to say that many, perhaps the majority of articulation disorders, do not reflect delays or deviations in articulation learning. As discussed early in the chapter, however, the acquisition of a behavior, such as speech articulation, requires adequate feedback. If a child has a deficiency in oral sensory awareness and discrimination ability it seems reasonable that such an impairment might well interfere with normal articulation learning.

There is currently a growing body of research that suggests that *oral stereognosis* (the ability to discriminate and identify objects and sensations in the mouth) is related to articulation disorders. *Oral form discrimination* testing has been the primary method of study. Although testing protocols have varied, there are two paradigms that have been widely employed. The first involves form recognition. A small three-dimensional geometric form is placed in the client's mouth and he is asked to manipulate the form orally and then to identify the form by pointing to its visually displayed counterpart. Typically, ten forms have been employed and error scores are expressed in percentages. A second procedure has been to place two objects in the client's mouth, one at a time, and then ask for a "same or different" judgment. Differences in the type and number of forms used, test protocols, and specific tasks have made the results of many investigations somewhat difficult to compare. (For discussions of test differences the interested reader is referred to works by Ringel, 1973; Torrans and Beasley, 1975; and McNutt, 1977).

Despite the disparity in procedures used by different investigators, it would appear that there is a positive relationship between oral form discrimination ability and defective articulation. A number of studies reveal such a relationship in both children and adults and for clients with both obviously organic impairment, as well as, for those with apparently "functional" articulation defects (Locke, 1968; Ringel, Burk, and Scott, 1968; Ringel et al., 1970, Moser; LaGourgue, and Class, 1967).

The study by Ringel, Burk, and Scott (1968) demonstrates not only a general relationship, but reveals a positive, rather monotonic relationship between the severity of the articulation defect and the degree of impairment in oral form discrimination ability. Lock (1968) demonstrates that children with good oral form discrimination scores are better able to learn non-English phonemes than those with poorer discrimination scores. This would certainly support the hypothesis that impaired oral sensory abilities in children may be causally related to retarded or deviant articulation learning. Sommers and Kane (1974), speaking of oral sensory awareness and the importance of kinesthetic feedback, state that it "helps an individual develop an awareness of muscle tensions and articulator positions at the moment speech sounds are produced and is thus important in the first stages of speech learning."

Another method of assessing oral stereognosis, although less frequently employed, is *difference limen* testing using two point discrimination procedures. The typical procedure involves the use of a caliper or forceps with uniform points and/or a calibration screw that permits adjustment and millimetric measurement of the distance between the two points. Usually multiple measures are taken at various locations in the oral cavity (tongue, lips, palate, etc.). The mean distance between the two points at which the client can no longer resolve or distinguish the two as separate stimulations is accepted as the difference limen (DL).

Both ascending and descending methods have been employed. Small DLs are interpreted as reflecting a greater degree of sensitivity and tactile discrimination ability than DLs of larger magnitude. It has been demonstrated that the tongue (especially the tip and apex) has smaller DLs than the lips or soft palate, suggesting a higher degree of sensitivity in this anatomical region (Ringel, 1973). This, of course, corresponds nicely to the finer adjustments, coordinations, and posturing required of the tongue tip and apex for production of linguaalveolar and linguadental consonants.

Although the research using two point discrimination has generally been less conclusive or consistent than the oral form discrimination research, there is some evidence to suggest that certain clients with articulation defects have poorer sensitivity (larger DLs) than others (Ringel, 1970; McNutt, 1977). However, there are indications that two point discrimination and oral form discrimination testing may not be measuring the same thing and require different levels of information processing. While the two would appear to be related, the degree of correlation is unknown. Studies that have employed both measures with the same subjects have reported somewhat different results (McNutt, 1977; Williams and LaPoint, 1971).

Part of the reason for the lack of consistency in findings probably relates not only to the difference in test procedures but also to the subjects studied. For example, it has been reported more than once that children who misarticulate the /r/ sound have poorer oral stereognostic ability than children who misarticulate other phonemes (Aungst, 1965; Weinberg, 1967; McNutt, 1977). McNutt also suggests that the severity of the articulation defect may also be a factor. Undoubtedly, additional research is needed to better determine the relationship.

Another approach to determining the importance of oral stereognostic abilities to speech articulation has been the experimental use of *nerve block anesthesia.* Although varying results have been reported, the general effect of oral sensory nerve block on the speech of normals, as summarized by Putnam and Ringel (1976), is a mild distortion primarily affecting the labial and anterior tongue consonants. This type of somesthetic deprivation in adults appears to result in perceptible distortion errors, but speech intelligibility is generally maintained. Putnam and Ringel speculate that speech might be more significantly affected, but that the individual appears to compensate for the inadequate sensory information by possibly reorganizing articulation efforts and using other muscles, less affected, to produce the critical sounds.

The nerve block anesthesia studies have been criticized for at least two reasons. Some have maintained that any attempt to block the afferent sensory nerve component will typically involve some spillover to the motor component producing some degree of paresis and that pure sensory deprivation is difficult, if not impossible to obtain (Harris, 1970; Putnam and Ringel, 1976). The second limitation involves the fact that such studies have little information value concerning the possible affects of prolonged deprivation on articulation learning in childhood. Further, with the possible exception of clients who suffer from significant, typically observable, neurologic disease, total anesthesia of a given oral region is probably not representative of the more subtle sensory-perceptual deficits that might be present in the majority of articulation defective clients. However, the research does suggest that kinesthetic feedback is important and necessary in the maintenance of articulatory accuracy.

In summary, the preceding would suggest that at least some clients with "functional" articulation defects have orosensory discrimination deficits. It has also been suggested that many clients with motor speech disorders (dysarthria, apraxia of speech) suffer from deficits in orosensory discrimination, at least at moderate and severe levels of the disorders (Aten, Johns, and Darby, 1971; Rosenbek, Wertz, and Darley, 1973; Haynes et al., 1977). A number of articulation therapy approaches include training exercises designed to improve or assist the client in compensating for orosensory perceptual disturbances. In light of the fact that some, possibly many, clients with articulation defects have associated or causally related oral astereognosis, fairly routine assessment of orosensory perception would seem justified.

FINE MOTOR SKILLS AND DIADOCHOKINESIS

Speech as a motor process requires the ability to execute rapid repetitive movements of the articulators. Of all behaviors, speech articulation is probably the most complex and requires extremely fine motor skills. It is probably for this reason that many have speculated on the possible relationship between articulatory proficiency and motor ability.

The early research is rather equivocal. A number of studies report finding a relationship between articulation proficiency and motor skills while others report generally negative results (Bilto, 1941; Albright, 1948; Reid, 1947; Prins, 1962). Following a review of the literature, Winitz (1969) suggests that there is insufficient evidence to support the theory of a relationship between articulation defects and general motor skill retardation. However, as Sommers (1974) suggests, the disparity in reported findings may well be due to the different definitions of "motor skills" and the differences in the tests employed by various investigators.

Taken as a whole, it would appear that those studies that have employed tasks involving *fine motor* skills have reported finding a relationship while those using test batteries consisting of largely *gross motor* skill activities have failed to demonstrate a significant correlation. According to Nicolosi, Harryman, and Kresheck (1968), fine motor skills pertain to "skillful, discrete, spatially oriented movements requiring use of small muscle sets, as in speech and the grasping and use of small objects." Gross motor skills are defined as those "pertaining to movements of large refined muscles for activities such as locomotor and balance."

Since speech articulation is unquestionably a fine motor skill, it is not surprising that defectiveness might correlate with other fine motor skill areas, such as eye-hand coordination, but not with gross motor ability. Clinical experience tells us that most children with "functional" articulation defects do not have apparent difficulty walking or maintaining balance control.

In two separate studies the Oseretsky Tests of Motor Proficiency (containing a number of fine motor skill subtests) has been administered to articulation defective elementary school aged children. Jenkins and Lohr (1964) examined thirty-eight first graders with severe articulation defects and compared their performances on the Oseretsky Test with thirty-eight normal speaking first graders. The children with articulation defects revealed significantly poorer motor skill development. Dickson (1962) suggests that articulatory defective children's motor skills (as indicated by the Oseretsky) may be of prognostic significance. Articulation tests and the Oseretsky were administered to articulatory defective kindergarten, first grade, and second grade children at the beginning of the school year. None of the children received speech therapy. At the end of the school year their articulation was again tested. Dickson reports that a comparison of test scores revealed that those children who no longer presented articulation errors had scored significantly higher on the Oseretsky than those who retained some of their sound misarticulations. These data would tend to suggest that children possessing reasonably normal fine motor skills might be expected to outgrow their articulation errors, at least to a greater extent than those with poor fine motor skills, given that all other factors are equal.

Quite naturally, the oral motor skills of speech defective individuals have also been investigated. It seems quite obvious that an individual must possess articulatory mobility adequate to support the extremely fine neuromotor adjustments and coordinations needed for speech production. The most common method of assessment, both clinically and experimentally, has been through the measurement of *diadochokinetic syllable rate.* Diadochokinesis refers to an individual's ability to rapidly start and stop the movement of the articulators and to execute repetitive, alternating, sequential movements typically associated with speech articulation.

Since the syllable is a basic unit of speech and is of convenient size and flexibility, rate of syllable production is frequently used as an index of diadochokinetic ability. There are two methods of assessment in wide use today. Both typically involve having the client repetitively produce, as rapidly as possible, single syllables such as /pʌ/, /tʌ/, and /kʌ/, bisyllables, such as /pʌtʌ/ and /tʌkʌ/, and trisyllable combinations, such as /pʌtʌkʌ/. The first method involves having the client produce as many repetitions as possible in a set period of time, say five or ten seconds, and then recording the number. This procedure, of course, requires that the examiner pay attention to both a stop watch and the number of repetitions at the same time. Of course this problem might be reduced by tape recording the task and counting the number of repetitions later (this is probably the only realistic way to obtain an accurate count).

A seemingly less cumbersome method has recently been proposed by Fletcher (1972). In Fletcher's "time-by-count" method, the client repeats a fixed number of syllables (twenty mono-, fifteen bi-, and ten tri-syllables) and the total time required to complete the repetitions is taken as the index of diadochokinetic ability. Fletcher published a table of normative data for children at different age levels that provides means and standard deviations. Thus, the examiner may compare his client's time with that of the "average" child at a given age level. It should be mentioned, however, that, although Fletcher provides standard deviation information, cutoff scores concerning "adequate" diadochokinetic ability are unavailable and, thus, speech pathologists are left to their own clinical experience and discretions in making judgments about what is and is not an adequate time score. In other words, how far below the mean must a child be before his diadochokinetic ability is no longer sufficient to support normal speech? The question is badly in need of investigation.

Another question in need of researching involves the use of nonsense syllables. It has been my experience that the use of nonsense syllables with young children, especially below the age of five or six, is difficult, and frequently the obtained results are of questionable validity. Some have suggested the use of real words, such as "patti-cake," "bubblegum," or "park-the-car" to obtain a more valid index of alternate motion rate in young children. This would seem like a more reasonable task for three to six-year-old children and might well provide an index more consistent with their actual diadochokinetic ability (McKelvey, 1977).

There can be no question that diadochokinetic ability is related to articulation defectiveness in certain populations. For example, children and adults with dysarthria have articulation defects that are directly and obviously attributable to the motor paralysis of the bulbar musculature. Hixon and Hardy (1964) demonstrate that the degree of speech defectiveness could be predicted with a fair degree of accuracy in cerebral palsied children by examining diadochokinetic information. Although the relationship is less obvious, studies also suggest that individuals with functional articulation defects have poorer oral motor skills than those with normal speech (Albright, 1948; Fairbanks and Spriestersbach, 1950; Prins, 1962; McNutt, 1977).

It has been suggested that both severity and articulation error types may well be differentially related to varying degrees of diadochokinetic impairment, although the issue is far from clear and needs further investigation. McNutt (1977) examined two groups of children: those who misarticulated the /r/ and those with /s/ misarticulations. Both were found to have poorer diadochokinetic rate scores than a matched group of normals. While McNutt did not find any significant differences between the /s/ and /r/ defective groups' diadochokinetic performances, he reports that the two groups differed in orosensory ability and suggests that further research with focus on severity and consistency of errors might well be revealing of fine oral motor skill differences as well.

The current focus by many scholars and clinicians concerned with articulation disorders would appear to be on the child's failure to acquire the phonological features of our sound system and the rules governing their correct usage. While this is certainly appropriate and, unquestionably, has added to our understanding of defective speech, we should not lose sight of the fact that nonfunctional disturbances in sensorimotor processing may well lie at the heart of the problem. Such nonfunctional differences may be the primary culprit underlying articulation learning problems or, at least, partially contributing factors. There seems to be little doubt that adequate sensory feedback and articulomotor control are vital to the child's articulation learning and development. The variables of auditory discrimination, orosensory perceptual skills, and oral fine motor skills are related to defective articulation in some clients. In order to further our understanding of these relationships we must continue our research efforts. It is important that we differentially identify those subgroups having such deficiencies so that we can plan and implement appropriate intervention strategies.

REFERENCES

Albright, R.: The motor abilities of speakers with good and poor articulation. *Speech Monograph, 15:*286-292, 1948.

Aten, J., Johns, D., and Darley, F.: Auditory perception of sequenced words in apraxia of speech. *J Speech Hear Res, 14:*131-143, 1971.

Aungst, L.: *The Relationship Between Oral Stereognosis and Articulation Proficiency.* Unpublished doctoral dissertation, Pennsylvania State University, 1965.

Aungst, L. and Frick, J.: Auditory discrimination ability and consistency of articulation of /r/. *J Speech Hear Disord, 29:*76-85, 1964.

Beasley, D., Shriner, T., Manning, W., and Beasley, D.: Auditory assembly of CVC's by children with normal and defective articulation. *J Comm Dis, 7:*127-133, 1974.

Berlin, and Dill: The effects of feedback and positive reinforcement on the Wepman Auditory Discrimination Test scores of lower class Negro and white children. *J Speech Hear Res, 10:*384-389, 1967.

Bilto, E.: A comparative study of certain physical abilities of children with speech defects and children with normal speech. *J Speech Dis, 6:*187-203, 1941.

Blasdell, R. and Jensen, P.: Stress and word position as determinants of imitation in first language learning. *J Speech Hear Res, 13:*193-202, 1970.

Cohen, J. and Diehl, C.: Relation of speech-sound discrimination ability to articulation-type speech defects. *J Speech Hear Disord, 28:*187-190, 1963.

Dickson, S.: Differences between children who spontaneously outgrow and children who retain functional articulation errors. *J Speech Hear Res, 5:*263-271, 1962.

Fairbanks, G.: Systematic research in experimental phonetics: a theory of the speech mechanism as a servosystem. *J Speech Hear Disord, 19:*133-199, 1954.

Fairbanks, G. and Spriestersbach, D.: A study of minor organic deviations in functional disorders of articulation. *J Speech Hear Disord, 15,* 1950.

Farquhar, M.: Prognostic value of imitative and auditory discrimination tests. *J Speech Disord, 26:*342-347, 1961.

Fletcher, S.: Time-by-count measurement of diadochokinetic syllable rate. *J Speech Hear Res, 15:*763-770, 1972.

Gammon, S., Smith, P., Daniloff, R. and Kim, C.: Articulation and stress/ juncture production under oral anesthetization and masking. *J Speech Hear Res, 14:*271-282, 1971.

Hardcastle, W.: *Physiology of Speech Production.* New York, Acad Pr, 1976.

Harris, K.: Physiologic measures of speech movements: EMG and fiberoptic studies. In *proceedings of the workshop: speech and the dentofacial complex. ASHA Reports, 5:*271-282, 1970.

Haynes, S., Johns, D., Richardson, S., and May, E.: Orosensory perception and apraxia of speech. *Texas J Audiology and Speech Pathology, Vol. 11, No. 3,* 1977.

Hixon, T. and Hardy, J.: Restricted motility of the speech articulators in cerebral palsy. *J Speech Hear Disord, 29:*293-306, 1964.

Jenkins, E. and Lohr, F.: Severe articulation disorders and motor ability. *J Speech Hear Disord, 29:*286-292, 1964.

Knaffle, J.: Auditory perception of rhyming in kindergarten children. *J Speech Hear Res, 16:*482-487, 1973.

Lenneberg, E.: *Biological Foundations of Language.* New York, Wiley, 1967.

Locke, J.: Discriminative learning in children's acquisition of phonology. *J Speech Hear Res, 11:*428, 1968.

Locke, J.: Oral perception and articulation learning. *Perceptual and Motor Skills, 26:*1259-1264, 1968.

McKelvey, J.: Performance of normal three and four year old children on ten selected oral motor tasks. *Texas J Audiology and Speech Pathology,* Winter, 10-12, 1977.

McNutt, J.: Oral sensory and motor behaviors of children with /s/ or /r/ misarticulations. *J Speech Hear Res, 20:*694-703, 1977.

McNutt, J., Pelc, M., and Dayton, D.: The effect of force variations upon two point discrimination at selected oral sites. *ASHA Reports, 13:*532, 1971.

Mange, C.: Relationships between selected auditory perceptual factors and articulation ability. *J Speech Hear Res, 3:*67-74, 1960.

Marquardt, T. and Saxman, J.: Language comprehension and auditory discrimination in articulation deficient kindergarten children. *J Speech Hear Res, 15:*382-389, 1972.

Menyuk, P.: The role of distinctive features in a child's acquisition of phonology. *J Speech Hear Res, 11:*183, 1968.

Menyuk, P. and Anderson, S.: Children's identification and production of /w/, /r/, and /l/. *J Speech Hear Res, 12:*39-53, 1969.

Monin, L. and Huntington, D.: Relationship of articulatory defects to speech sound identification. *J Speech Hear Res,* 352-366, 1974.

Moser, H., LaGourgue, J., and Class, L.: Studies of oral stereognosis in normal, blind and deaf subjects. In Bosma, J. (Ed.): *Symposium on Oral Sensation and Perception.* Springfield, Thomas, 1967.

Nicolosi, L., Harryman, E., and Kresheck, J.: *Terminology of Communication Disorders.* Baltimore, Williams & Wilkins, 1968.

Perozzi, J. and Kunze, L.: Relationship between speech sound discrimination skills and language abilities of kindergarten children. *J Speech Hear Res, 14:*382-390, 1971.

Powers, M.: Functional disorders of articulation. In Travis, L. (Ed.): *Handbook of Speech Pathology.* New York, Appleton-Century-Crofts. P.-H., 1957.

Prins, T.: Motor and auditory abilities in different groups of children with articulation deviations. *J Speech Hear Res, 5:*161-168, 1962.

Putnam, A. and Ringel, R.: A cineradiographic study of articulation in two talkers with temporarily induced oral sensory deprivation. *J Speech Hear Res, 19:*247-266, 1976.

Reid, G.: The etiology and nature of functional articulation defects in elementary school children. *J Speech Hear Dis, 12:*143-150, 1947.

Ringel, R.: Oral sensation and perception. In Wolfe, W. and Goulding, D. (Eds.): *Articulation and Learning.* Springfield, Thomas, 1973.

Ringel, R.: Oral sensation and perception: a selective review. In *speech and the dentofacial complex: the state of the art. ASHA Reports, 5:*188-206, 1970.

Ringel, R., Burk, K., and Scott, C.: Tactile perception: Form discrimination in the mouth. *British J Discord Comm, 3:*150-155, 1968.

Ringel, R., House, A., Burk, K., Dolinsky, J., and Scott, C.: Some relationships between oral sensory discrimination and articulatory aspects of speech production. *J Speech Hear Disord, 35:*3-11, 1970.

Ritterman, S.: The role of practice and the observation of practice in speech sound discrimination learning. *J Speech Hear Res, 13:*178-183, 1970.

Rosenbek, J., Wertz, R., and Darley, F.: Oral sensation and perception in apraxia of speech and aphasia. *J Speech Hear Res, 16:*22-36, 1973.

Reid, G.: The etiology and nature of functional articulation defects in elementary school children. *J Speech Hear Disord, 12:*143-150, 1947.

Schwartz, A. and Goldman, R.: Variables influencing performance on speech sound discrimination tests. *J Speech Hear Res, 17:*25-32, 1974.

Shelton, R., Johnson, A., and Arndt, W.: Delayed judgment speech sound discrimination and /r/ or /s/ articulation status and improvement. *J Speech Hear Res, 20:*704-717, 1977.

Sherman, D. and Geith, A.: Speech sound discrimination and articulation skill. *J Speech Hear Res, 10:*277-281, 1967.

Sommers, R. and Kane, A.: Nature and remediation of functional articulation disorders. In Dickson, S. (Ed.): *Communication Disorders: Remedial Principles and Practices.* Glenview, Scott, Foresman, 1974.

Sommers, R., Meyer, W., and Fenton, A.: Pitch discrimination and articulation. *J Speech Hear Res, 4:*56-60, 1961.

Sommers, R., Meyer, W., and Furlong, A.: Pitch discrimination and speech sound discrimination in articulatory defective and normal speaking children. *J Auditory Res, 9:*45-50, 1969.

Spriestersbach, D. and Curtis, J.: Misarticulation and discrimination of speech sounds. *Q J Speech, 37:*483-491, 1951.

Stitt, C. and Huntington, D.: Some relationships among articulation, auditory ability, and certain other variables. *J Speech Hear Res, 12:*576-594, 1969.

Tannahill, J. and McReynolds, L.: Consonant discrimination as a function of distinctive feature differences. *J Auditory Res, 12:*101-108, 1972.

Torrans, A. and Beasley, D.: Oral stereognosis: effect of varying form set, answer type and retention time. *J Psycholinguistic Res, 4,* 1975.

Travis, L. and Rasmus, B.: The speech sound discrimination ability of cases with functional disorders of articulation. *Q J Speech, 17:*217-226, 1931.

Van Riper, C.: *Voice and Articulation.* Englewood Cliffs, P-H, 1958.

Weinberg, B., Liss, G., and Hollis, J.: A comparative study of visual, manual, and oral form identification in speech impaired and normal speaking children. In Bosman, J. (Ed.): *Second Symposium on Oral Sensation and Perception.* Springfield, Thomas, 1970.

Weiner, P.: Auditory discrimination and articulation. *J Speech Hear Disord, 32:*19-28, 1967.

Wepman, J.: *Auditory Discrimination Test.* Chicago, Language Research Associates, 1958.

Wepman, J.: *Relationship of Auditory Discrimination to Speech and Reading Difficulties.* Paper presented at the annual convention of the American Speech and Hearing Association, 1959.

Winitz, H.: *Articulatory Acquisition and Behavior.* New York, Appleton-Century-Crofts, 1969.

Williams, W. and LaPoint, L.: Correlations between oral form recognition and lingual touch sensitivity. *J Percept Motor Skills, 32:*840-842, 1971.

CHAPTER 3

Articulation Development

C HILD DEVELOPMENT involves cognitive, locomotor, social, and linguistic learning. While all four are indentifiably separate areas there is little doubt that they are interrelated and, to varying degrees, interactive processes. However, it is the latter of these, language development, that is of immediate concern and, more specifically, the phonological component of such development.

When a child first comes into the world he finds himself bombarded with an array of stimuli that at first must seem somewhat nonsensical and devoid of meaning. Developmentally, his primary task would appear to involve pattern recognition, placing events in order and discerning meaning from the apparent chaos. In other words, he must establish a relative understanding of the world around him so that he can learn to function adequately in it.

THE NATURE-NURTURE QUESTION

The nature-nurture question has been debated for years. It is of both theoretical and clinical relevance to the speech pathologist. The question concerns itself with the relative importance of the child's biology (nature) as opposed to his environment and learning (nurture) in the process of phonological acquisition and development.

Some contend, and there is a good deal of evidence to support the position, that the newborn comes into the world phylogenetically "prewired" or predisposed to acquire speech and language behavior. This *nativist* position suggests that speech is a species specific trait in humans, much as flight is a species specific trait and predetermined behavior in birds. The nativists contend that the human infant's biological structure and neurophysiology are selectively adapted and designed for the acquisition of speech (McNeill, 1970) and point to the close

69

correspondence between neurophysiological and structural maturation (readiness) and the emergence of the behavior (Lenneberg, 1967). The suggestion is that in the absence of significant sensory, structural, or neurophysiological defects, and with simple exposure to speech and language, the behavior will be incorporated in the child's repertoire and will become manifest as biological "readiness" and maturation dictate. The position places only limited importance on the traditional concepts of environment and "learning."

Support for the nativistic position may be drawn from the infant speech perception research as reviewed in Chapter 1. Studies employing heart rate and high amplitude sucking dishabituation paradigms have pretty convincingly demonstrated that young infants do indeed discriminate between various places of articulation and voicing phonological features. These data would certainly suggest some inborn ability to detect rather subtle differences in the speech code.

Additional evidence for the "nature" position may be drawn from the apparent linguistic universality of speech development. It would appear that regardless of country, culture, or the child's specific native language, speech development proceeds with a rather remarkable similarity in chronology and with certain landmarks being obtained at roughly equivalent ages. In light of the wide range in child raising practices and the differences in phonologies across countries, it is rather surprising that most children universally go through the same temporal sequence of babbling, lallation, echolalia, and begin using "true speech" at approximately one year of age. In her 1968 study, Menyuk found that American and Japanese children's phonological development follow the same chronology with reference to distinctive feature acquisition and usage. The fact that speech development is universally similar would certainly offer support for the nativists' argument of biological predisposition.

However, on the other side of the coin is the "nurture" or *empiricist* philosophy that suggests that human behavior, including phonological, is learned through experience and interaction with the environment. In its extreme form, the philosophy suggests that the newborn child is like a "blank slate" and that all behavior is a direct result of environment, parent raising practices, and learning experiences. Most of those who adhere to the empiricist position do not hold to this extreme view. However, they do believe that environment plays a more important role than biology in the child's development.

A number of studies demonstrate that both vocal and verbal behaviors are subject to the principles of classical and operant learning. A series of studies with two and three month old infants demonstrate that vocal behavior can be increased by contingently applied, positive social consequences and that positive human interaction with infants is necessary to achieve the increase (Rheingold, Gewirtz, and Ross, 1959; Weisberg, 1963; Todd and Palmer, 1968). These studies are important in that they demonstrate vocal behavior to be susceptible to operant conditioning principles and show that the mere presence of an unresponding adult is not sufficient to increase vocal "play" in infants.

There is probably no single theory of vocal development that embodies the empiricist philosophy to a greater extent than *Mowrer's Autism Theory.* According to Mowrer's (1952) Theory, vocal development occurs as a process of classical conditioning and stimulus generalization. Basically, the Theory proposes that since mothers frequently talk to their infants while administering primary care (feeding, removing soiled diapers, etc.), mother's voice assumes secondary reward value through repeated contiguous association with the primary care, which has inherent reward value (classical conditioning). Then, since the infant's vocalizations are acoustically similar to mother's (similar stimuli) they assume some of the strength of mother's vocalizations in signalling that the conditions are present for primary reward (stimulus generalization). In this manner, the infant's vocal behavior assumes reward value and, being pleasurable, increases.

From this theory we might conclude that children talked to while being fed and cared for should exhibit more imitative babbling than children not talked to during the administration of primary care. We might also assume that those sounds produced by the infant that are more like mother's will tend to increase while those unlike mother's and outside of the native language would tend to decrease in frequency (stimulus-response gradient — see Winitz, 1969). This is exactly what appears to happen as the child's vocalizations become more language specific during the purported lallation and echolalic stages of vocal development.

Many of those who adhere to the empiricist philosophy suggest that verbal and meaningful articulatory behavior is acquired through a process of operant learning (Skinner, 1957; Winitz, 1969). It has been suggested that as the child's vocalizations become increasingly language specific, his phonetic strings will begin to approximate "real words." Although such productions may at first be accidental, the parents interpret them as meaningful and reinforce them. Supposedly the "string" occurs often enough and is sufficiently reinforced to increase and become a part of the child's repertoire of behaviors. It is suggested that at first the parents' standards are rather lax and that reinforcement is given for any word approximation. However, with time, the parents' standards are increased and articulatory behavior develops as a process of selective reinforcement, stimulus, and response generalization and with extinction of articulatory behavior that is not reinforced.

It would appear that both the empiricist and nativistic positions have foundation and contain some inherent "truth." The more current thinking by many professionals in the child development areas is that neither position is completely correct nor totally in error. Both biology and environment are considered important. There seems to be little doubt that the ability to acquire speech is indeed a species specific trait. Despite rigorous efforts to teach subhuman primates to talk, little success has been reported. It would appear that our human biology is designed in a way that is special, and, in that sense, acquisition of the behavior is biologically predetermined. It would also appear that we have special neural mechanisms that allow us to process speech and extract the rules underlying its organization and usage. However, if speech development was totally attributable to biological predeterminism and physical maturation then defective speech would occur only as sequelae to sensory, structural or neurophysiological impairment.

This would not appear to be consistent with clinical experience. I have frequently been amazed by children who have rather severe structural or neurological defects and rather good articulation skills. I have also worked with many children who possess apparently normal structures and an adequate sensorium and neurology, but who, nevertheless, present rather severe articulation problems. To the author at least, this suggests that the child's environment and learning experiences are important variables in speech development. The very fact that speech therapy is effective with many articulatory defective children suggests that environment and learning experience are potentially influential.

Part of the argument between the nativists and empiricists may be definitional. How the terms *teaching* and *learning* are defined would seem to be important to the discussion. I have maintained for some time that parents do not teach speech and children do not learn to talk in the traditional manner in which we use the terms. I do not know of any mother, or speech pathologist for that matter, who possesses sufficient knowledge and ability to literally "teach" her child the processes of speech. Few parents possess a knowledge of articulatory physiology and, even if they had sufficient knowledge, the young child would hardly be able to comprehend the instructions.

However, children do learn to talk if by *learn* we mean that the child acquires the behavior, at least in part, through experience and interaction with his environment. Mothers do teach speech if by *teach* we mean that they provide a speech model and environment conducive to articulation learning. However, based on the fact that most children (approximately 95%) develop speech normally and are free of articulation defects, we must conclude that the range of acceptable environments is quite wide. A child's ability to learn speech is apparently quite tolerant of environmental variation and, in some cases, poor maternal teaching. While maternal modelling and imitation-reinforcement are undoubtedly important and involved in the child's acquisition of articulation skills, their exact role in the process and degree of importance are unclear (Rees, 1975). What does seem clear is that the young child has the sensorimotor abilities necessary to produce a wide range of possible sounds that resemble the phonemes present in most languages. It also seems clear that the developing child's sound productions progressively become more language specific and that, gradually, his somewhat ambiguous productions of phonemelike sounds develop into purposive linguistic units, providing him with a repertoire of "building blocks" for meaningful expression.

As Templin (1973) suggests, the processes underlying the production of phonemes in words is quite different than those involved in the production of a sound that to the listener resembles a phoneme. She states that "the production of a sound in a word involves not only motor control, but perceptual discrimination and cognitive processing, whereas the babbling utterance may be largely a sensorimotor function" (p. 55). It may be that the child's biology provides him with a species specific sensorimotor and, to a certain degree, perceptual system capable of speech development and production. However, only through environmental interaction is he able to "learn" the specific features and rules inherent in his native phonology and through production experience (practice) and feedback he is able to establish closed loop control of articulation.

DEVELOPMENTAL COMPONENTS OF ARTICULATION

With the advent of modern phonological theory we have come to realize that articulation development involves more than a mastery of the motor movement patterns necessary to produce speech sounds. For years we considered speech sound development only in this manner. As such, our focus was on the child's *phonetic* development and we interpreted normative data as reflecting the age levels at which a child was expected to master the motor acts underlying correct *production*. When we consider the child's phonetic development our attention is primarily on *performance*.

However, articulation development involves more than learning the articulomotor aspects of production. In fact, as previously discussed, children below the age of three years are generally able to execute the necessary movement sequences needed to produce all of the phonemes of English and frequently demonstrate the sounds in nonmeaningful or inappropriate contexts. Undoubtedly, phonetic learning continues beyond this age and a child must learn the necessary coarticulation skills involved in the production of meaningful linguistic sequences. Certainly it is important to continue asking "how" a child is able to master the rather intricate processes of speech production. However, with the evolution of distinctive feature theory (see Chapter 1) and the theory of generative phonology (Chomsky and Halle, 1968), it has become clear that we must also seek to understand what underlies such development. We must ask questions concerning the child's developmental phonological *competence,* i.e. the developmental knowledge of the sound system that makes performance (speech production and perception) possible.

We can only make inferences about a child's phonological competence at a given age through experimental observations of his performance. Because we have been studying this aspect of articulation development for only a short time, we are less comfortable with our theories of such development than with those concerning phonetic development. However, it would appear that the developing child must acquire a conceptual understanding of our sound system before he can participate, at any relative level of sophistication, as a speaker-listener. He must acquire a discriminative-conceptual repertoire of the minimally contrastive elements (distinctive features) that make meaningful differentiation among the phonemes of our system possible and he must learn the rules that govern the correct combination and usage of such features in building the phonemes of his community language. While a number of researcher-clinicians have referred to this aspect of development as "phonological" (Crocker, 1969), the term is widely used to denote both the phonetic and phonemic aspects of articulation. Therefore, following the lead of Winitz (1969), I have chosen, as have others, to use the word *phonemic* to refer to this aspect of development.

Thus, the acquisition of articulation skills requires the development of both the phonemic conceptual and phonetic articulomotor components of the behavior.

An analogy may help to clarify the two components. We might liken the task of the young infant in acquiring articulation skills to that of a naive observer trying to make sense out of a ball game that he is exposed to for the first time. Without any prior knowledge of the game and with no one to provide him with instruction, his initial observations of the activity on the field may lead him to conclude that the game is confusing, without apparent purpose and devoid of meaning. However, with repeated exposure to the game he realizes that there are always the same number of players on the field. He also begins to discern the fact that each of the players is somewhat different, i.e. they consistently assume a set position on the playing field.

Likewise, our young child develops an awareness that there are a finite set of features in his community language and that they are distinctive. As our naive observer continues to receive repeated exposure to the game he also comes to realize that the players can interact with each other in only a limited number of ways and have specific roles to play (in football the center cannot move down the field and receive a pass but the end can). In other words, he begins developing an understanding of the rules governing the interaction of the players in completing plays. He observes that these rules are always followed and enforced. Similarly, our developing child learns that there are a finite number of rules governing the interaction and combination of features in forming phonemes. Likewise, these rules are also enforced in that violation results in his not being understood by those in his environment.

As our observer becomes more sophisticated, he discerns that certain combinations of plays result in scores while others result in failure. The child also develops an understanding that certain phoneme combinations are permissible and result in higher linguistic units while others do not, e.g. /sk/ is a permissible combination while /zk/ is not.

Following attendance at an extremely large number of games, our observer develops a rather high level of competence. His knowledge of the players and the rules of the game with all its nuances is fairly sophisticated. He then decides that he wishes to participate, to play the game himself. However, despite his relatively high level of competence he finds that his performance leaves much to be desired. With a great deal of practice, however, he develops a reasonable facility at playing the game. He also discovers that in playing the game himself he has acquired additional knowledge of some of the fine points.

Our observer's developing knowledge of the game is obviously analogous to the child's phonemic development. His learning to participate and play the game is like the child's phonetic development of speech. Of course the analogy is not completely accurate in many respects. It should be obvious that in the child's articulation development the phonemic and phonetic components progress together in more of a parallel fashion. A child does not wait until he has a complete phonemic mastery before beginning to develop phonetic skills. In fact, phonetic experimentation and learning probably facilitates phonemic development. For example, the child's ability to fully conceptualize the phonemes /f/ and /θ/ probably requires a phonetic awareness of the rather subtle difference between the two in terms of place of articulation obtained through phonetic practice and kinesthetic monitoring.

The interaction between the phonetic and phonemic systems in articulation development is just beginning to be explored. The issue is a complex one and the questions are not easily answerable. Even the relative age(s) of mastery of the two components is unclear. It would seem that phonemic development both influences and is influenced by the child's morphological and syntactic development. Winitz (1969) suggests that the bulk of phonemic development is complete by the age of three years, with further articulatory refinements being the result of "(1) morphological development, (2) sound acquisition in words, and (3) mastery and refinement of certain motor units" (p. 74).

Others suggest that phonetic and phonemic development progress together to full mastery of articulation skills. It would appear that most children below the age of three years do indeed possess the ability to both discriminate among and produce all of the phonetic features in their community language, at least in isolation or in linguistically irrelevant or inaccurate contexts. However, as Crocker (1969) suggests, phonemic (phonological) development involves the child's increasing ability to appropriately select and combine the features, by rule, into higher order linguistic units. Crocker suggests that the developmental mastery of sounds may be accounted for by rule learning and that those sounds that are learned later in the child's development involve more complex feature combinations and more difficult attendant rules.

It seems reasonable to suggest that phonemic development

continues well past the age of three years with mastery of the developmentally more advanced phonemes requiring the acquisition of more complex feature selection and combinatorial rules. It would also appear to be consistent with clinical observations of normally developing children's sound substitution errors.

Most of these age-appropriate errors involve the substitution of a phoneme that is different from the target phoneme by only a single feature (Menyuk, 1968). In many instances these errors appear despite the fact that the child may well produce the feature (attribute) correctly in other phonemes requiring it. This would certainly suggest a phonemic rule problem and since these errors may be observed normally in children past the age of three years, we must conclude that phonemic development continues past this age. Another example may be found in the child who consistently substitutes one sound for another, say f/θ, but nevertheless produces the target sound correctly when attempting to produce a different phoneme, for example θ/s. Thus, a child may say "fumb," "baftub," and "teef" but also demonstrate the ability to produce a correct /θ/ when saying "the thun ith in the thky." Obviously the error is not a phonetically based one, but rather reflects a phonemically based rule problem.

It is reasonable to assume that phonetic and phonemic development proceed together up to the age of approximately five or six years. Some additional phonetic learning may be required after this age in order for the child to master the complex articulomotor sequences needed in the production of certain consonant clusters. Certainly this is speculative and the exact role and importance of the phonetic and phonemic systems in the child's later stages of articulation development are unclear. The picture is complicated by the fact that the developmentally more advanced phonemes not only require more complex feature combinations but are also motorically more difficult to produce.

In 1941, Jakobson suggested that phonemic development involves the child's acquisition of sounds on the basis of phonetic categories (English translation, 1968). According to his theory the child first acquires those sounds that are maximally contrastive (labial stop versus open back vowel) and then developmentally learns to differentiate among and produce phonemes that have progressively less decided phonetic feature differences (nasals versus orals, dental versus labial consonants, etc.). Along somewhat similar lines, Menyuk (1968) suggests that those features that American and Japanese children acquire first have the most decided on and off (+, −) characteristics and are the easiest to discriminate (see Chapter 1). It would appear that those phonemes that are acquired earliest by the developing child are the easiest to produce motorically but, of equal or possibly greater significance, contain distinctive features whose attributes are perceptually maximally contrastive and, therefore, easiest to discriminate.

In 1969, Crocker proposed a competence-based model of phonological development in which he specified the rules that the child must master in order to combine features and feature sets into recognizable phonemes. Crocker demonstrates that his model is able to account for the progressive appearance of phonemes in the child's phonemic development, according to existing normative data. His model is also able to predict the normal sound substitution errors that occur in the developing child's speech. According to the model, once the child has mastered the "primary features" of his community language (those required to establish and distinguish among the primary phonemic classes or groups of sounds) and has learned to combine these into "prime feature sets" (early sound production), development is largely a process of mastering the combinatorial or recombinatorial rules that make the production of more specific (intraphonemic) phonemes possible. Referring to this stage of development, Crocker states, "the subject, then, may be said to acquire not the features as such, not the sound as such, but rather the hypothesized rules for the manipulation of the features to form the feature sets which previously had not appeared in his developing phonological system" (p. 206). While Crocker's model appears to be consistent with our observations of the child's developmental mastery of the sound system, he suggests interpretive caution and the need for research validation.

Crocker's model suggests that a delay in the child's articulatory development may be due to either of two things: (1) an unsuccessful early attempt to combine features into sets upon which later sound development is predicated or (2) faulty rule learning involving developmentally more advanced phonemes requiring complex feature combinations.

McReynolds and Huston (1971) examined ten children with severe articulation defects and subjected their sound errors to a distinctive feature analysis. They conclude that feature errors are consistent across phonemes and that a single feature error may account for multiple phoneme errors. They suggest that errors occur as the result of either a feature being absent from the child's repertoire or the inappropriate use of a feature (inappropriate rule application).

In 1972, Pollack and Rees suggested that articulation errors may reflect phonetic, articulomotor execution problems that occur secondary to physiological or orofacial defects or they may represent phonemically based, developmental deviations in the child's acquisition of the rule system. In the latter case, they refer to the child's defective articulatory behavior as an "ideolect" that reflects, not a simple, immature, delayed phonemic development but, rather, a deviant and typically consistent rule system. This obviously has significant implications for evaluating, classifying, and treating children with articulation defects.

A topic of concern to both the phonetic and phonemic components of articulation development is *generalization*. The fact that generalization is important in articulation learning has been repeatedly demonstrated in the therapy room. For example, in children who misarticulate the /s/ and /z/ phonemes, correction of the defective /s/ will more frequently than not result in an improvement in the child's ability to produce the /z/ as well. In this case we say that generalization has occurred across phonemes with similar stimulus characteristics. Similarly, a child who is taught to produce a sound correctly in one word or context may also demonstrate an ability to produce the sound correctly in nontrained words or contexts. Along these lines, McReynolds and Bennett (1972) demonstrate that when distinctive features were taught in selected nonsense syllable contexts (initial and final positions) correct use of the features appeared in nontrained contexts and in previously defective phonemes that were not worked on in therapy. As a matter of fact, they report a 69 to 84 percent decrease in the overall occurrence of the feature errors. This obviously reflects a significant amount of generalization. Undoubtedly, generalization is an extremely important part of the normal child's articulation development.

As we have said, phonemes are comprised of sets of distinctive features. Distinctive features are phonemic concepts just as words are semantic concepts. Just as a child generalizes and gradually learns the limits of semantic concepts, he must do likewise with distinctive features in the process of articulation development. A specific analogy at the semantic level may help to clarify the point. During the child's first year he may begin to drink out of a cup. He identifies the stimulus dimensions of "his" cup. It may be blue, small, have an opening at the top, a handle on the side and hold his milk. By repeated association he learns that this object is called *cup*. At first, only his cup is so labelled. However, with only a little exposure to other representatives (exemplars) of this class of objects, he generalizes to all other objects with similar stimulus dimensions.

At this point the child has developed a concept of *cupness*. He may, of course, initially overgeneralize. For example, his concept of cupness may well include any object from which one drinks, including glasses. Gradually, however, he learns the limits and permissible contexts and functions of the concept. He learns that objects that are typically taller than cups, generally transparent, and usually devoid of handles are labelled *glass* and that cups have a somewhat different function, e.g. hold less liquid and are used for different drinks, such as coffee.

Similarly, the child must develop a concept of distinctive features, e.g. voiceness, nasality, frication, etc. However, somewhat unlike semantic development and the association between the word and a given exemplar, the child hears and learns to discriminate between the presence and absence of a given feature in a number of phonemes. Undoubtedly, though, some generalization is required, and inherent in the process is "rule learning," possibly as suggested by Crocker. Although, the exact manner in which a child learns to combine a given feature with all other appropriate feature sets to produce all the phonemes requiring the presence of the feature remains somewhat unclear.

At the phonetic level, it has been assumed that, once a child has learned to produce a phoneme correctly in one context, he will generalize the correct motor movements and posturing to other contexts that are phonetically similar. However, while generalization as the result of facilatory contexts (stimulus generalization) undoubtedly occurs, a recent study by Elbert and McReynolds (1978) suggests that other variables may be more important. They report that a child's stimulability (ability to produce the sound correctly under imitative conditions) is more predictive of the amount of generalization that will occur than specific context information. They suggest that generalization begins once the child is able to imitate the sound correctly and that this reflects his development of the correct "articulatory concept." It is obvious that additional study of articulatory concept development, generalization, and stimulability at various age levels would indeed be warranted and might shed considerable light on our understanding of articulation development.

DEVELOPMENTAL NORMS

The chronological development of the sound system is remarkably orderly. Despite some slight variation from child to child, the ages at which certain phonemes and phoneme types emerge in the speech of children is generally consistent. A series of studies by Orvis Irwin in the 1940s, as reviewed by Winitz (1969), has shed a good deal of light on the chronological development of the sound system during both the vocal and verbal stages of evolution. Irwin studied ninety-five infants from birth to two and one-half years of age. He and his associates tape recorded unelicited, spontaneous samples of the children's vocalizations and verbalizations at two-month intervals and transcribed the samples using the International Phonetic Alphabet (IPA).

Although Irwin has been criticized for employing phonemic transcription methods with obviously nonphonemic, preverbal vocalizations, his data nonetheless provide us with valuable information concerning the emergence and frequency of usage of particular sound and phoneme-types during the early ages of development. Irwin's data revealed that the one to two-month-old infant's vocalizations primarily consist of seven phoneme types, with a high frequency of occurrence of glottals, velars, and midvowels. Until about the age of six months, the infant produces more vowels than consonants with the frequency of back vowels increasing with age. Labial and linguadental consonants, according to Irwin, begin to appear with some consistency in the five to six-month-old with a corresponding drop in the occurrence of glottals. The nine to ten-month-old demonstrates a wide range of consonant types and most consonants are present by twenty months. By thirty months of age the percentages of time that given consonants appear in the child's speech begins to approximate the adult ratios. Irwin's data also suggest that by thirty months children are able to produce practically all of the English phonemes. However, this does not suggest that they are using them in a linguistically relevant or error-free manner. It simply means that the sounds have appeared in the child's speech. Obviously it takes longer for the child to integrate these articulatory gestures into meaningful and appropriate contexts in their community language.

Irwin's studies were concerned primarily with establishing the ages at which sounds and phonemes appeared in the developing child's speech. Other studies have focused their attention on phoneme mastery. Although there has been some consistency across studies, at least in terms of very general chronology of sound mastery, significant differences have been reported concerning the age at which children master a specific phoneme.

Undoubtedly, part of the reason for the disparity lies in different investigator's definition of *mastery* and the different age ranges of the children sampled. For example, in normative studies by Wellman et al. (1931), Templin (1957), and Prather et al. (1975) age of mastery is defined as the minimum age at which 75 percent of the children sampled could produce the phonemes correctly in various positions of single words. On the other hand, studies by Davis (1938) and Poole (1934) report the ages at which 100 percent of the subjects correctly articulated the phonemes.

While such developmental normative data are valuable we must be cautious in our interpretation and clinical applications of the information. For example, it is obvious that such data do not necessarily give us an index of the age at which the average child is able to correctly articulate a given phoneme. Rather, they provide information concerning the mean age at which 75 or 100 percent of the children master a phoneme. These rather stringent criteria may have resulted in an age inflation relative to the "average" child. The use of a 50 percent criteria with reported means and standard deviations might provide more valuable clinical information.

Another problem with such data is that testing has typically been done at the word level only. A child may well be able to articulate a given phoneme correctly in an isolated word but not have mastered it in spontaneous, connected speech. However, within the scope of these limitations, the data may be useful in making general decisions concerning age-appropriate articulation ability.

Table III below summarizes the Templin (1957) and Prather et al. (1975) data. While it can be seen that there is general

TABLE III

AGE, IN YEARS AND MONTHS, REFLECTING MASTERY OF CONSONANT PHONEME PRODUCTION ACCORDING TO STUDIES BY TEMPLIN (1957) AND PRATHER ET AL. (1975)

Phoneme	Templin	Prather, et al.
p	3-0	2-0
m	3-0	2-0
n	3-0	2-0
h	3-0	2-0
ŋ	3-0	2-0
d	4-0	2-4
k	4-0	2-4
f	3-0	2-4
w	3-0	2-8
b	4-0	2-8
t	6-0	2-8
g	4-0	3-0
s	4-6	3-0
r	4-0	3-4
l	6-0	3-4
ʃ	4-6	3-8
tʃ	4-6	3-8
ð	7-0	4-0
ʒ	7-0	4-0
v	6-0	4+*
θ	6-0	4+*
z	7-0	4+*
dʒ	7-0	4+*

*Phoneme not produced correctly by 75 percent of children at upper age level of study.

agreement relative to the chronology of phoneme mastery, there are obviously significant differences between the reported age mastery levels. Prather et al.'s data suggest phonemic mastery at much earlier ages than that of Templin or the earlier studies. Although Templin did not include two-year-old children in her study, Prather et al. were unable to suggest a viable reason for the disparity in age mastery levels for phonemes above the three year level.

It can be said that there is almost twenty years separating these two studies and even a greater distance between the Prather et al. study and the others mentioned above. Some suggest that the times are different and that contemporary children may indeed be more precocious in sound development than children growing up twenty, thirty, or forty years ago. Some have pointed to the possible influence of concentrated exposure to television and the electronic media to account for such an hypothesis. Although modern influences may have some effect, I personally doubt that they can fully account for the disparity in reported findings. Regardless of the reason(s), however, my personal experience with children tells me that the Prather et al. data are more accurate. Their data are limited by the fact that they did not include children above the four year level in their study.

As Sander (1972) suggests, probably a better and clinically more utilitarian way to express phoneme acquisition data is in terms of relative ranges of mastery. As Darley (1978) suggests, "we are less likely to misunderstand the process if we think of it as encompassed within definable ranges rather than encapsulated in absolute numbers." Sander presents the data from previous studies in this manner as do Prather et al. in expressing their own findings. In both cases, the ranges of mastery for each phoneme included the earliest ages at which 50 to 90 percent of the children correctly articulated the sound. Using the same criteria, I have pooled the data from the studies by Wellman et al., Templin, and Prather et al. The age ranges in which 50 to 90 percent of the children, across the extremes of the three studies, correctly produce each of the consonants are listed in Table IV. The ages at which 50 percent of the children are able to correctly produce the respective phonemes is felt to more accurately reflect the average child's age of mastery.

TABLE IV

AGES AT WHICH 50 AND 90 PERCENT OF CHILDREN CORRECTLY PRODUCE
CONSONANT PHONEMES

Phoneme	50% Criterion	90% Criterion
n	2-0*	3-0
m	2-0*	3-0
p	2-0*	3-0
h	2-0*	3-0
t	2-0*	6-0
k	2-0	4-0
f	2-0*	4-0
w	2-0*	3-4
ŋ	2-0*	6-0
b	2-0*	4-0
g	2-0	4-0
s	2-0	8-0
j	2-4	4-0
d	2-0	4-0
l	2-8	6-0
r	2-8	6-0
ʃ	3-0	7-0
tʃ	3-0	7-0
dʒ	3-0	7-0
v	3-4	8-0
z	3-6	8-0
ʒ	3-8	8-0†
ð	4-0	8-0
θ	4-0	7-0

*Mastered by 50% of children below reported age level.
†Not mastered by 90% of children at oldest age level studied.

By scanning the list in Table IV we can derive a general picture of the chronology of phoneme mastery. It is interesting to note that by four years of age the average child, according to these data, is able to correctly produce all the consonant phonemes. However, it is also apparent that complete mastery by many children does not occur until eight years of age. This tends to suggest a rather wide variability. Examination of these data will also reveal that the greatest age ranges (differences between the 50 and 90% criteria) occur for the phonemes that are typically acquired later in the developmental sequence. For example there is a four to four and one-half year mastery range for the phonemes /ʃ/, /tʃ/, /dʒ/, /v/, /z/, /ʒ/, /ð/, with a six year range for /s/. It is interesting that these phonemes, together with the /θ/ and semivowels /r/ and /l/ are the most frequently misarticulated by children. It can be noted that these phonemes consist of seven fricatives, two affricates and two semivowels. There is no question that they require finer motor control and more exact articulatory posturing for accuracy of production than those acquired at earlier ages. They also require the incorporation of more difficult to discriminate distinctive features and more complex combinatorial rules.

From the data in Table IV we can see that by the close of second grade 90 percent of all children are correctly articulating 80 percent of the consonant phonemes and that by eight years of age all the consonants have been mastered. Thus, employing these very lenient criteria as a definition of normal limits, we may conclude that any consonant misarticulations after the age of eight can no longer be considered developmentally normal and merit speech therapy. Of course, a consideration of the need for therapy and whether or not a specific child's articulatory deviations are age-appropriate requires an examination of the specific sound errors.

Certain sounds are expected to be mastered earlier than others and developmentally "normal" errors typically have certain characteristics. For example, age-appropriate errors typically involve the substitution of an earlier acquired phoneme for one acquired later in the developmental sequence. More commonly the error production is in the same phonemic class as the target phoneme and substitution errors are more common than omissions or distortions. Also, such misarticulations typically involve only single distinctive feature errors (Menyuk, 1968). Some of the most common developmental sound substitutions are: θ/s; ð/z; j/l; w/l; w/r; f/θ; s/θ; t/θ; d/ð; v/ð; s/ʃ; t/tʃ; ʃ/tʃ; d/dʒ; θ/f; v/f; b/v; t/k; g/d; w/j; and l/j.

While the developmental data are far from absolute and more research is needed, they do provide us with a general index by which to judge the appropriateness of certain sound errors in a child at a given age. Of course, other considerations are important in making therapy decisions and prognostic estimations. For example, Templin (1973) suggests that "as a whole, children who have many misarticulations in pre-kindergarten are likely to continue to have misarticulations into fourth grade." Thus, in addition to the particular phonemes in error and the nature of the errors, we must also consider the number of misarticulations in making clinical decisions. Other variables, such as the child's stimulability and the consistency of the error(s), are also important.

REFERENCES

Chomsky, N. and Halle, M.: *The Sound Pattern of English.* New York, Har-Row, 1968.

Crocker, J.: A phonological model of children's articulation competence. *J Speech Hear Disord, 34:*203-213, 1969.

Darley, F.: Appraisal of articulation. In Darley, F. and Spriestersbach, D.: *Diagnostic Methods in Speech Pathology.* New York, Har-Row, 1978.

Davis, I.: The speech aspects of reading readiness. 17th Yearbook of the Department of Elementary School Principals. *NEA, 17:*282-289, 1938.

Elbert, M. and McReynolds, L.: An experimental analysis of misarticulating children's generalization. *J Speech Hear Res, 21:*136-150, 1978.

Jakobson, R. (English translation by A. Keiler): *Child Language, Aphasia, and Phonological Universals.* The Hague, Mouton Pr, 1968.

Lenneberg, E.: *Biological Foundations of Language.* Cambridge, MIT Pr, 1967.

McNeill, D.: *The Acquisition of Language.* New York, Har-Row, 1970.

McReynolds, L. and Bennett, S.: Distinctive feature generalization in articulation training. *J Speech Hear Disord, 37:*462, 1972.

McReynolds, L. and Huston, K.: A distinctive feature analysis of children's misarticulations. *J Speech Hear Disord, 36:*155-166, 1971.

Menyuk, P.: The role of distinctive features in children's acquisition of phonology. *J Speech Hear Res, 11:*138-146, 1968.

Mowrer, O.: Speech development in the young child: 1. The autism theory of speech development and some clinical applications. *J Speech Hear Disord, 17:*263-268, 1952.

Pollack, E. and Rees, N.: Disorders of articulation: some clinical applications of distinctive feature theory. *J Speech Hear Disord, 37:*451, 1972.

Poole, I.: Genetic development of articulation of consonant sounds of speech. *Elem Eng Rev, 11:*159-161, 1934.

Prather, E., Hedrick, D., and Kern, C.: Articulation development in children aged two to four years. *J Speech Hear Disord, 40:*179-191, 1975.

Rees, N.: Imitation and language development: issues and clinical implications. *J Speech Hear Disord, 40:*339-350, 1975.

Rheingold, H., Gewirtz, J., and Ross, H.: Social conditioning of vocalizations in the infant. *J Comp Physiol Psychol, 52:*68-73, 1959.

Sander, E.: When are speech sounds learned? *J Speech Hear Disord, 37:*55-61, 1972.

Skinner, B.: *Verbal Behavior.* New York, Appleton-Century-Crofts, 1957.

Templin, M.: *Certain Language Skills in Children.* Institute of Child Welfare Monograph Series, No. 26. Minneapolis, U of Minn Pr, 1957.

————: Developmental aspects of articulation. In Wolfe, W. and Goulding, D. (Eds.): *Articulation and Learning.* Springfield, Thomas, 1973.

Todd, G. and Palmer, B.: Social reinforcement of infant babbling. *Child Dev,* *39:*591-596, 1968.

Weisberg, P.: Social and nonsocial conditioning of infant vocalizations. *Child Dev, 34:*377-388, 1963.

Wellman, B., Case, I., Mengert, I., and Bradbury, D.: Speech sounds of young children. *University of Iowa Studies in Child Welfare.* Iowa City, U of Iowa Pr, 1931.

Winitz, H.: *Articulatory Acquisition and Behavior.* New York, Appleton-Century-Crofts, 1969.

CHAPTER 4

Articulation Disorders

A RTICULATION DISORDERS typically command more of the speech pathologist's time and attention than any other single disorder of speech. It is estimated that 5 percent of all school-aged children have articulation defects of sufficient magnitude to warrant professional attention. For speech pathologists working in the public schools, children with defective articulation generally constitute 75 to 80 percent of the caseload. The total percentage may be even higher if we consider children who have defective articulation secondary to hearing loss, cleft palate, cerebral palsy, and in association with generalized language retardation. Darley (1978) estimates the figure to be around 90.5 percent. It seems clear that an understanding of the nature of articulation disorders is of paramount importance to the practicing speech pathologist, regardless of employment setting.

A child with an articulation defect may not be able to talk clearly enough to be understood by those around him or, even if his speech is basically intelligible to most listeners, it may draw attention to the child and result in a negative reaction or perception by others. The effects of such disorders may include the genesis of feelings of inadequacy in the child, problems in peer interaction, and problems in social and emotional development. Such children also frequently show poorer achievement records during the early school years. Many children with articulation disorders seem to have difficulty in learning to read and in mastering the language arts. Although in the minority, articulatory defective children show a higher incidence of specific learning disability than children free of articulation impairment. It seems clear that the disorder may have a significantly deleterious affect on the individual and should not be taken lightly.

ETIOLOGICAL CONSIDERATIONS

The importance of determining, if possible, the cause or causes of an articulation defect cannot be over stated. It must be remembered that speech disorders, including that of articulation, are present in only a small minority of the population; they are the exception, not the rule. Given a normal brain, a reasonably responsive sensorium, an intact structural mechanism, and, seemingly, a modicum of positive stimulation and a child will develop speech normally. Defective speech is then indicative of some kind of underlying problem.

The etiology or cause of the articulation defect may be a single underlying disturbance in biology or environment or it may result from a number of relatively minor disturbances that, in combination, prevent the individual from acquiring normal facility. In this respect, an articulation disorder is symptomatic of an underlying disturbance. To treat the symptom (articulation defect) without an understanding of the underlying problem may result in an inappropriate or inefficient program of remediation and frustration for the client and clinician as well.

By analogy we might consider an individual with a fever who goes to a physician seeking medical assistance. The underlying pathology may be a systemic infection of some type. However, if the physician in his assessment examines only the presenting symptoms (fever, malaise, etc.) and does not diagnose the underlying pathology, his treatment may be restricted to prescribing an alcohol rub to bring down the fever and aspirin to relieve the discomfort. While the patient may feel better, the odds are that the symptoms will recur. On the other hand if the physician diagnoses the underlying problem and prescribes the appropriate antibiotic the chances for successful therapy have been substantially increased.

Of course the analogy is far from perfect. Obviously speech pathologists do not treat medical pathologies. Some may even contend that there is little we can do about the underlying cause(s) of the speech defect even if identified, so why bother. However, the fact of the matter is that our approach to therapy, as well as prognosis, will be affected by the etiology. Speech therapy is, for the most part, compensatory. Through it we provide clients with an intensified learning environment, hopefully one that is facilatory, and we use techniques designed to help the client compensate for an underlying deficiency that prevents him from acquiring the skills naturally. In therapy we may also directly improve certain underlying deficiencies, such as selected discrimination problems. It seems clear then that if we are to assist the client to compensate for a given condition or to work on improving it directly, we must first be able to identify it.

Many children may have rather minor, subtle deviations in biology or environment and yet develop articulation skills within broad normal limits. Articulation impairment may occur when a child is unable to compensate for a significant single deviation in biology or environment or, probably more commonly, multiple coexisting deviations. Factors that are known to contribute to or to be causative of articulation impairment include structural abnormalities of the speech mechanism, neuromotor disturbances, neuroperceptual impairments, mental retardation, hearing loss, and certain severe deviations in the child's environment during the critical speech learning years.

The classification of an articulation disorder as *functional* in etiology is probably the single most common diagnosis made by speech pathologists. The term is generally used to denote faulty learning due to environmental influences. The term *dyslalia* is occasionally used to designate such disorders. While the classification of an articulation disorder as functional may occasionally be justified, the diagnosis is typically abused. It is a diagnosis commonly made by default. The speech pathologist typically classifies the disorder as functional when unable to find any obvious organic pathology. However, the fact is that there are frequently no likely environmental candidates for the role of causative culprit either. Thus, the label has come to mean "no obvious organic impairment."

In such cases, probably the majority of those classified as functional, the use of the term *idiopathic* would perhaps be more appropriate. The term suggests a disorder of unknown etiology. I suspect that many such disorders are the result of subtle, coexisting, factors that lie beneath the clinical eye of the speech pathologist. It is probably also true, as Van Riper and Irwin (1958) discuss, that organic disturbances earlier in the child's development may have caused the problem but may no longer be present. Of course this may be equally true of disturbing environmental influences. Faulty articulation, in such cases, may be maintained by habit strength and may be quite resistant to correction in the older child or adult.

Prior to discussing some of the apparent causes of articulation disorders a few words of caution seem to be in order. Frequently, following the identification of a major etiological factor, such as structural deformity, the client's total articulation errors are attributed to the defect. This may be a significant clinical mistake. Many of the client's misarticulations may be unrelated to the defect. It is important to examine for all possible disruptive factors even though one may be obvious and also to keep in mind that certain errors may be due to faulty learning while others may well be attributable to some structural or neurophysiological limitation. It should also be remembered that clients are individuals and may be differentially affected by a given condition. I have seen children with almost identical degrees of orofacial defectiveness where one has developed astonishingly good articulation skills and the other has very poor speech. Thus, the degree of influence of a given etiological factor can never be stated with absolute certainty.

Structural Abnormalities

Structural abnormalities of the speech mechanism may underlie a number of articulation disorders. Perhaps the most obvious and potentially disruptive are clefts of the palate and lip. Although there are individual exceptions, the severity of the associated articulation disorder typically corresponds to the severity and magnitude of the orofacial deformity. It is reasonable to expect a more severe articulation problem in a client with a congenital, bilateral, complete cleft palate and lip than in a client with a partial cleft of the soft palate only and no lip involvement. The articulatory error pattern will also vary depending, at least partially, on the structural defect.

While the problems are typically multiple, two major factors generally account for the articulation disorders in such clients. The first concerns the fact that, despite early surgical repair, the oral environment may not be adequate for normal articulation learning. In such cases, the child may develop inappropriate sound substitution errors in compensation for his inadequate mechanism. Articulation errors such as glottal for oral stop plosives, pharyngeal for oral fricatives, and posterior plosives, frequently coupled with glottal stops, for anterior plosive and fricative phonemes may well evolve in this manner. Unable to produce the correct oral plosives and fricatives the child may attempt to compensate by producing substitute sounds that are the best acoustic approximations he can make. Unfortunately, such errors become an integral part of the child's phonetic repertoire. Even if subsequent surgery provides the child with a normal oral structure the errors typically persist and are difficult to correct in speech therapy.

The second major problem concerns the structural-physiological limitations involved in the client with an orofacial cleft. Even in cases where the client has learned the sounds correctly (for instance, correct place of articulation), productions may be distorted due to an inadequate anatomy and physiology.

There is an impressive amount of research that suggests that the primary reason for disturbed articulation in cleft palate children is an inadequate velopharyngeal mechanism (Spriestersbach and Powers, 1959; Subtelney and Subtelney, 1959; Hardy and Arkebauer, 1966; Van Demark, 1966; and others). Inability or inefficiency in closing off the nasopharyngeal port through velopharyngeal contact results in a loss of air pressure through the nasal cavity and an inability to generate sufficient oral air pressure to produce the plosive, fricative, and affricate phonemes. As a result, these phonemes are frequently omitted or severely distorted in clients with cleft palates. Other problems that may underlie articulation errors in cleft palate and lip clients include the following: (1) dental deviations that further interfere with accurate fricative production; (2) lip involvement, such as immobility due to scarring, which may interfere with the normal articulation of labial consonants; and, (3) frequent, recurring middle ear infections (otitis media), which may well interfere with normal articulation learning. Spriestersbach and Sherman (1968) provide an excellent indepth review of the speech disorders found in children with palatal clefts.

Although not nearly as prevalent as the lay community might think, *ankyloglossia* or *tongue-tie* does indeed occasionally present itself and may cause articulation impairment. The condition typically involves a congenitally short lingual frenum that may anchor the anterior tongue to the floor of the mouth. In addition to being excessively short, the frenum may also extend anteriorly more than usual with the tongue tip having a slight v-shaped indentation. McEnery and Gaines (1941) report finding four cases in 1000 children.

Generally, if the tip and apex of the tongue can contact the alveolar ridge without mandibular effort, the condition need not concern the speech pathologist. However, if the tongue tip cannot be raised above the level of the lower incisors and cannot be protruded interdentally the condition may well interfere with normal speech production. The most commonly defective sounds in such a condition are the /r/, /l/, /t/, /d/, /θ/, /ð/, /s/, and /z/. Many of these children may develop rather elaborate compensatory modes of production. For instance, the /r/ and /l/ phonemes may be produced with only the tongue blade elevated, the /t/ and /d/ via apicoalveolar contact and the /s/ and /z/ with the tongue tip in the down position. Of course these sounds are frequently distorted.

The decision concerning whether or not the frenum should be surgically clipped must be made by the child's physician. However, it is not uncommon for the physician to ask the speech pathologist for advice relative to the degree of influence the ankyloglossia is having on speech development. Although it is a rather simple surgery, typically requiring only an office procedure, complications may occur. For example, scar tissue may build up following surgery. However, in my experience such complications are rare and the potential benefit in cases like that described would seem to warrant the surgical intervention. Of course, speech therapy is still generally needed in order to teach the client how to produce the error sounds correctly once he has the lingual mobility to do so and to extinguish the compensatory error patterns that frequently are present.

Dental problems constitute structural deviations frequently believed to be a cause of articulation impairment in certain clients. Likely candidates include malalignment of the upper and lower teeth (malocclusion), missing teeth (edentulous space), jumbled or individually malaligned teeth, and openbite. A number of researcher-clinicians report a relationship between defective articulation and dental abnormalities (Huber and Kopp, 1942; Kessler, 1954; Snow, 1961; Bankson and Byrne, 1962; Fymbo, 1936, and others).

The particular effect of a malocclusion on speech will depend upon the type and severity of the malalignment and, of course, upon the individual client's susceptibility to such deviations. This last point is important since it is clear, from clinical experience, that many children with rather substantial malocclusions develop normal speech or show no signs of associated articulation errors. Malocclusions may occur in the form of overbites (distoclusion), underbites (mesioclusion), end to end bites (neutroclusion), and crossbites.

The most frequent malocclusion associated with articulation impairment is an overbite, sometimes referred to as an overjet. In such a condition the upper teeth distend anteriorly away from the lower, making correct production of the /s/, /z/, /θ/, /ð/, /ʃ/ and /ʒ/ phonemes difficult. In extreme cases, the bilabial phonemes /p/, /b/ and /m/ may be produced with a compensatory lower lip to upper teeth contact. Productions of the /f/ and /v/ phonemes may be made only with effort or compensatory movement in both severe cases of overbite and underbite. The specific effects of such compensatory movement patterns on other phonemes in connected speech are unknown but probably vary substantially from individual to individual.

An occlusal anomaly that frequently occurs concomitantly with overbite is openbite. In such a condition the anterior teeth do not approximate in the superior-inferior dimension and errors with the linguadental and labiodental fricatives are quite common. The most frequent errors associated with openbite, as well as with missing front teeth, are /θ/ and /ð/ substitutions for /s/, /ʃ/, and /z/, /ʒ/, respectively. Such an error pattern is referred to as a frontal or interdental *lisp*. It is believed that such malocclusions may result from either excessive and protracted thumb sucking during childhood or from *tongue thrust* (reverse swallow). In tongue thrust the deviate swallowing pattern, as the name implies, involves an anterior thrusting of the tongue against the anterior teeth, sometimes protruding interdentally. The chronic pressure may force the upper teeth upward and outward. Winitz (1969) provides an excellent summary of the topic. Malalignment of individual teeth may result in a deviation of the air stream and consequent distortion of the fricative phonemes.

It is common for children to lose their incisors during the transition from deciduous to permanent teeth, typically during the first and second grades. As a result the /s/, /z/, /ʃ/ and /ʒ/ phonemes may be misarticulated. These sounds may be only slightly distorted or a /θ/ or /ð/ may be substituted for them. In such cases the speech pathologist is often uncertain as to whether therapy is warranted. Some maintain that the errors will prove self-correcting with the eruption of the permanent teeth. It has been the author's experience that the decision should be based on the specific articulatory tongue postures used to produce the phonemes. If the place of articulation is correct but the sounds are distorted because of the missing teeth, speech therapy is probably best postponed for later consideration after the permanent teeth have erupted. However, if the tongue actually protrudes between the arches in the form of a true frontal lisp, therapy is generally indicated.

It is not uncommon for clients who have had recent orthodontic work to experience some articulation difficulty associated with newly introduced braces, dentures, or prosthetic devices in the mouth. However, in the author's experience, such difficulty is typically of brief duration and the client soon compensates for the modifications in the oral cavity. Thus, the articulation errors are generally transient, lasting no more than a week or two. If they should persist, short-term speech therapy is usually effective in assisting the client to compensate.

There are a host of other structural deviations involving the speech mechanism which may contribute to articulatory defects, however, their frequency of occurrence is sufficiently small to preclude extensive discussion. Conditions such as facial and lingual clefts, microglossia and macroglossia, mandibular deformities, and complete or partial aglossia may well cause an articulation disorder. The speech pathologist must assess each case individually and based on a knowledge of physiological phonetics determine the potential contribution of a given structural defect to the client's articulation disorder.

Neuromotor Disturbances

As previously stated, speech is a highly complex fine motor skill. Articulation requires higher level, cortical planning and sophisticated fine motor execution. As such, the process requires a reasonably intact central and peripheral nervous system. For speech the critical components of the system include the following: (1) an area of the left cortex in the frontal lobe, known as Broca's Area, which is believed to be responsible for the recall and organization of the motor commands that are necessary to produce a given articulation; (2) an area of the cortex, both left and right, known as the "motor strip," which contains large motor neurons capable of initiating motor impulses; (3) the pathway or tract, known as the "cortico-bulbar" tract, which conveys the neuromotor impulses to the brain stem; (4) a system of nuclear masses deep in the cortex through which the cortico-bulbar tract passes, known as the basal ganglia, which assist in maintaining appropriate muscle tone and in modifying the neural impulses; (5) motor neurons in the brain stem; and, (6) the cranial nerves (V, VII, IX, X, XI, and XII) that convey the impulses to the muscles of the head, neck, and face and make movement of the articulators possible. Damage to any part of the system may result in an articulation impairment.

The particular kind and severity of the impairment will depend largely on the site of the lesion(s) and the degree of interruption of the system(s) affected. Damage to Broca's Area, described above, may result in an articulation impairment known as *apraxia of speech*. Damage to any of the other components or areas described (the motor system itself) may result in a *dysarthria*.

Dysarthria is a generic term that is used to designate any speech defect that occurs secondary to brain damage and that results from weakness, incoordination, or paralysis of the speech musculature. Thus, the term may be equally applicable to children with cerebral palsy and poststroke adults. The term is not specific only to articulation and, more often than not, there are associated disturbances involving respiration, phonation, and resonance. The particular type and amount of involvement of the basic speech processes will, again, depend upon the site of lesion. Darley, Aronson, and Brown (1969; 1975) describe six basic types of dysarthria: spastic, flaccid, ataxic, hypokinetic, hyperkinetic, and mixed. With training and clinical experience the speech pathologist may learn to discern the distinctive acoustic characteristics and specific speech (phonatory and articulatory) disturbances typical of each type of dysarthria. Depending on the type and particular speech processes involved, the symptoms may vary widely.

Respiration may be completely normal or may be affected to the point of being completely inadequate to support phonation. Voice quality may be weak, breathy, and hypernasal in flaccid dysarthria or may be harsh and periodically strained as in some cases of spastic dysarthria. Articulation disturbances may vary from the typically slow, labored patterns found in flaccid types to the frequently hurried "rushes" of blurred speech manifest by Parkinson's disease patients with hypokinetic dysarthria. While the symptoms vary widely, clients with dysarthria generally have problems with diadochokinesis, use of appropriate vocal intensity, maintaining and using appropriate pitch and pitch variation, and consistent articulation errors, typically consonant distortions and omissions. The consonants affected first are those that require more exact fine motor control, such as the affricates, fricatives, /r/, and consonant blends. The plosives may be affected in cases of velar paralysis.

Vowel distortions suggest a more severe motor disturbance and may appear in clients with moderate to marked dysarthria. In some clients, the paralysis or incoordination of the phonatory and articulatory musculature may be so severe that speech production is not possible. In such cases, the speech pathologist must be realistic. Although a trial period of speech therapy may be appropriate in questionable cases, the speech pathologist should be willing to consider alternate forms of communication (communication boards, etc.) for the client.

Apraxia of speech as a separate diagnostic entity has been widely recognized by members of the profession only during the last ten years or so. Foundation work on methods of differentially identifying the disorder from the dysarthrias was done by Shankweiler and Harris (1966) and by Johns and Darley (1970), the latter becoming a classic study for clinical reference. Although apraxia of speech frequently occurs together with dysarthria and aphasia, it may occur in isolation as well. It occurs in the absence of any weakness, paralysis, or incoordination of the speech musculature and is basically a disorder of the motor memory for speech articulation. As such, motor speech programming is impaired and the client has difficulty with the formulation of the neural commands and sequencing needed by the motor system to carry out correct articulatory expression. Unlike the dysarthric client, the articulation errors in apraxia of speech are highly inconsistent and the client's automatic speech is generally better than planned purposive speech attempts. The effects on speech may vary from slight articulatory impairment to a complete inability to produce speech in severe cases. The typical error pattern, as suggested by Darley and associates, includes the following: (1) substitution, omission, and additive, intrusive errors more commonly involving the fricative and affricate phonemes and consonant blends; (2) effortful groping and trial and error behavior on misarticulated phonemes; (3) articulatory substitutions that are not always motoric simplifications of the target phoneme; (4) greater difficulty on initial consonant sounds and on words having more than one or two syllables; (5) greater difficulty with imitative than with spontaneous speech; and, (6) difficulty with diadochokinetic syllable tasks that require alternate syllable productions.

A frequent accompaniment of apraxia of speech is *oral apraxia*. In such clients there is a reduced efficiency or complete inability to volitionally move the oral musculature in attempting nonspeech tasks, such as voluntarily phonating, protruding the tongue or pretending that they are performing such activities as licking an ice cream cone, blowing, whistling, etc. However, like apraxia of speech, the impairment occurs in the absence of motor paresis or incoordination and the nonspeech behaviors mentioned above may be accomplished normally by the client under automatic or reflexive conditions. Since a predominantly phonetic approach is recommended for clients with apraxia of speech, oral apraxia may significantly interfere with progress in therapy. As such, it is important for the speech pathologist to be cognizant of and to identify the condition in order to plan an appropriate therapy regimen.

While the concept of apraxic speech difficulty has been applied to the adult population for many years, its consideration as the culprit underlying articulation disturbances in children is just beginning to receive widespread attention. It has probably received considerably more attention in Europe than in the United States. However, Eisenson (1972) discusses the problem, and in a 1974 article, Yoss and Darley develop a criterion list for the differential diagnosis of "developmental apraxia of speech" from "functional" disorders of articulation.

In examining school-aged children with moderate to severe articulation defects they report finding approximately 50 percent with symptoms meeting the criteria for a diagnosis of developmental apraxia of speech. Interestingly, these children had previously been diagnosed as having functional impairments. The children had a high incidence of neurologic soft signs (generalized dyspraxia, poor motor control, awkwardness, etc.) and an inordinately high occurrence of oral apraxia. Their performances on diadochokinetic syllable tasks were significantly poorer than their nonapraxic counterparts. They showed great difficulty with multiple syllable words with errors of syllable omission, revision, and intrusive additions. Their individual articulation errors are reported to be more aberrant than those of other children with articulation disorders, containing two and three feature errors, more distortions, and inappropriate sound additions.

Experienced clinicians will recognize children in their caseloads who fit the above description and who seem to have problems with articulatory programming and sequencing. They will also recognize that such clients are often difficult to work with effectively and that traditional forms of speech therapy are frequently unproductive. These children merit special attention and, if Yoss and Darley are correct, may constitute a significant percentage of even the typical caseload. The topic will be discussed in greater depth later in the book.

The causes of neurogenic speech disorders are many and varied. The etiology may be vascular (CVA thrombosis, embolism, hemorrhage), neoplastic (brain tumor), infections (viral or bacterial invasion of the nervous system, such as meningitis, encephalitis), traumatic (head injury), degenerative (such as multiple sclerosis), toxic (such as carbon monoxide poisoning), or metabolic. Probably the most frequently presenting etiologies in adult clients are cerebrovascular accident (stroke) and head injury.

In children, the symptoms of dysarthria and apraxia are typically more clearly present in cerebral palsy. However, like the term *dysarthria, cerebral palsy* is not a specific diagnostic label. Rather it is a generic term that implies a nonprogressive brain damage that occurs in children prior to neurological maturation (the criteria generally include completion of the myelinization process around the ages of seven, eight, or nine). Thus, the condition may be congenital or acquired during or after birth. While the causes of cerebral palsy are numerous, the single factor that presents itself most frequently is anoxia (lack of sufficient oxygen supply to the brain). Extensive discussion of the topic would go beyond the purpose and scope of the book and there are numerous excellent texts available to the interested reader. It should be obvious by now that the particular type and severity of speech impairment (the particular type of dysarthria) will depend upon the site of lesion and the type of neuromotor disturbance.

There is no question that many children with cerebral palsy have severe articulation disorders. However, many do not. Mecham, Berko, and Berko (1966) report that 70 to 80 percent of cerebral palsied children have some type of speech difficulty. However, in a study by Achilles (1955), only 43 percent were reported to have "poor" articulation. As with any form of dysarthria, the consonants most severely affected are those requiring the most exact articulatory posturing and having inherent motoric complexity. However, caution should be exercised in attributing the articulation problems in cerebral palsy children exclusively to the obvious neuromotor disturbance. Children with cerebral palsy have a much higher incidence of sensory-perceptual deficits and mental retardation than those children who are not brain damaged. These and other factors may significantly contribute to a given child's articulation disorder.

Neuroperceptual Impairments

It is not uncommon for speech pathologists to spend many hours engaged in therapy designed to improve a client's auditory perceptual skills. Whether or not such practices are warranted with the majority of articulation impaired clients is debatable. However, it is clear that many clinicians consider auditory perceptual deficits to be at the heart of many articulation problems. In fact, probably the bulk of speech therapy approaches are auditorily based, although not necessarily designed to directly improve perceptual deficits.

As discussed in Chapter 2, there is a good deal of research that suggests a rather strong relationship between articulation impairment and defects in auditory discrimination ability. Those clients with mild or mild to moderate articulation disorders typically have difficulty in correctly identifying and discriminating only their error phonemes. In other words, they do not appear to have generalized auditory perceptual problems. In all probability their discrimination deficits are phonologically based and are related to the fact that these clients have not acquired an accurate "auditory image" of the specific error phonemes or have not developed an ability to phonetically differentiate between their error sounds and the correct phoneme. It is doubtful that these clients have neurogenic auditory processing deficits.

On the other hand, it has been demonstrated that clients with more severe articulation disorders (more than four separate phoneme errors with multiple feature errors and reduced speech intelligibility) tend to have generalized speech discrimination deficits, involving more than their error sounds and frequently demonstrate deficits in nonspeech auditory processing as well. In åddition to speech discrimination deficits, these clients have been reported to have problems involving pitch perception, auditory memory, sound blending, correctly identifying and retaining auditory sequential material, etc. It is suspected that many of these clients have auditory perceptual problems of a neurogenic nature.

Yoss and Darley (1974) report finding "auditory perception and auditory sequencing" disturbances in children with severe articulation disorders regardless of whether or not they evidenced characteristics of developmental apraxia of speech. Slorach and Noehr (1972) examined the auditory processing functions of dyslalic children using a dichotic listening test and an ordered recall paradigm. They report that, unlike normal children, the dyslalic children were not able to maintain a right ear advantage under the ordered recall task. They speculated that these children may "have difficulty in developing sufficiently strong neural trace patterns within the dominant hemisphere" of the brain. This would tend to suggest that the primary deficit lies with auditory sequential memory for speech in the left hemisphere. However, as stated above, many severe cases have problems with speech as well as nonspeech auditory stimuli and the basic disturbances may be generalized to a number of perceptual processes in addition to memory. On the basis of their findings, Slorach and Noehr suggest that "dyslalic children may have a true perceptual deficit related to the maturation of the auditory system" and that such a proposal is congruent with clinical experience and the observation that children with "functional articulation disorders are, in the majority of cases, known to improve with maturation." To the author, the hypothesis would appear to be tenable and such a deficit may well be the culprit underlying many of the articulation disorders we see clinically.

An immature central auditory system may also explain the observation that children with moderate and severe articulation disorders frequently evidence delayed language development as well. Such children show a much higher incidence of retarded vocabulary growth and syntactic disturbances (Shriner, Holloway-Sayre, and Daniloff, 1969). A neurologically immature auditory system might well result in both articulation and language deficits and might explain the significant correlation between the two.

Of course, a specific focalized lesion to the superior portion of the temporal lobe might also explain the findings of generalized auditory processing problems in many cases of severe articulation impairment. Such lesions may go undetected for the most part since the motor and association areas may not be affected. However, in severe cases either the magnitude of the lesion or criticalness of its location may be such that the child is totally unable to meaningfully segment and identify the salient acoustic characteristics of the waveform.

In such cases, both speech and nonspeech auditory stimuli are nonmeaningful to the child. We refer to such a condition as *auditory agnosia*. If the lesion is congenital or acquired early in the child's development, speech and language skills will not be acquired or, at the very least, will be severely defective. The fact that such children are able to process stimuli through the visual and tactile sensory modalities in seemingly a normal fashion is testimony to the fact that the lesion involves only the auditory system. Obviously most articulatory defective children do not have such severe auditory perceptual problems. However, in many cases we may be seeing the partial affects of a less severe lesion. Thus, either a focal temporal lobe lesion or a neurological immaturity in the growth of the auditory cortex may result in observable articulation impairment, language delay as well as secondary problems such as learning to read and write. It is the author's opinion that such neurogenic involvement may lie at the heart of many of the problems children have who are diagnosed as learning disabled.

As summarized in Chapter 1, auditory perceptual skills include an ability to segment the ongoing acoustic signal, identify the segmented units, store them in short-term memory and synthesize (blend) them into larger meaningful units. Difficulty with any one of these processes may have a deleterious effect on the entire system and may interfere with higher level association processes. As stated, children with severe articulation problems frequently have deficits in speech and nonspeech auditory discrimination and memory. Beasley et al. (1974) demonstrated that children with articulation disorders also may have deficits involving auditory synthesis. They examined the abilities of sixty articulatory defective first, second, and third grade children to assemble auditorily segmented syllables and compared their performances to sixty matched normal speaking children. They found the articulation impaired youngsters to be significantly inferior to the normal children in their ability to synthesize the isolated sounds into meaningful words. A similar study employing nonspeech sounds might provide valuable information relative to the specificity of the deficit.

Thus, children with moderate and severe articulation disorders show a high incidence of auditory perceptual deficits characterized by problems in discrimination, memory, synthesis, and, ultimately, correct auditory identification. As a general rule of thumb, those who have difficulty with both speech and nonspeech auditory stimuli probably have subtle neurogenic involvement. The two likely candidates are an immature central auditory system or a focalized temporal lobe lesion. On the other hand, clients with speech perception difficulty only, in the absence of other symptoms of brain damage, probably have linguistically based perceptual deficits.

Mental Retardation

Undoubtedly, there is a general consensus among practicing clinicians that mentally retarded children and adults show a much higher incidence of defective articulation and language delay than those with normal intelligence. As summarized by Winitz (1969), Powers (1971), and Darley (1978), although the correlation between articulation defectiveness and composite IQ scores is low for the general population, the relationship is strong for those with IQs below seventy. Thus, we might expect a high occurrence of articulation defects among the retarded with increasing speech defectiveness among the more severely retarded.

In a study by Wilson in 1966, 53.4 percent of 777 educable mentally retarded children evidenced defective speech. Those with lower mental ages had error patterns characterized by omissions and phonemic substitutions while those in the higher ranges tended to manifest primarily distortion type errors. Although there does not appear to be a single pattern of articulation defectiveness among the retarded, experience suggests that their errors are not completely like those of other clients with impaired articulation. They do appear to have the greatest difficulty with the phonemes that are normally acquired later in the developmental sequence. However, they also have a higher frequency of omission errors, especially final syllable omissions, than one might expect in nonretarded clients and they seem to have a greater incidence of vowel distortions, suggesting a more severe deviation. We must be cautious, however, in attributing all of their articulation problems to reduced intelligence. The incidence of sensory-perceptual and physiological deficits is generally higher in the mentally retarded population and suggests other possible contributing causes for the articulation defect. For instance, while their omission and substitution errors may well be attributable to phonemic learning deficiencies, the prevalence of distortion errors and general "oral inaccuracy" may be reflective of subtle sensorimotor deficits.

It should be remembered that many individuals who are classified as mentally retarded have relatively normal speech. However, as a general rule of thumb the lower the IQ and mental age equivalent, the greater the likelihood of speech impairment. Articulation defectiveness is practically universal among the severely retarded and, in the author's experience, those with IQs below approximately thirty may never develop oral-verbal skills at all. It should be remembered that speech articulation requires not only adequate sensorimotor skills but also an intellectual ability sufficient to conceptualize the abstract phonemic system and to master the rather complex phonological rules underlying the sound system. Undoubtedly, the major problems inherent in the mentally retarded child's slower development of speech and language skills are a reduced abstract conceptualization ability and a reduced ability to generalize from learned exemplars. While speech therapy can be effective in bringing about an improvement in these client's articulation skills, the above factors are probably to blame for the typically slower progress encountered by most clinicians.

Hearing Loss

The importance of normal hearing to the development of adequate articulation skills cannot be overstated. The young child's ability to hear the speech of others and, as discussed in Chapter 2, to monitor his own articulations through the auditory channel is essential to normal expressive speech development. Hearing loss has long been recognized as a critical and relatively frequent etiological factor underlying articulation disorders.

The specific effect of hearing loss on articulation will depend on the amount, type, and chronicity of the loss and the age of onset. Hearing losses that are acquired after speech and language skills have been mastered may have little effect on articulation. If the acquired loss is bilateral and severe there may be some change in speech over time, such as alterations in pitch and loudness with eventual consonant distortions or final consonant omissions. If the hearing loss is congenital in nature or acquired early during the child's critical speech learning years the effects on articulation will be much greater. With mild or mild to moderate auditory sensitivity impairments the consonants most affected will be those produced with the least intensity, i.e. the fricative and affricate phonemes. Since these are also predominantly comprised of high frequency energy components, individuals with moderate and even severe high frequency losses, but with reasonably good low frequency sensitivity, may manifest similar articulation difficulty.

As the hearing loss increases in severity other consonant phonemes may be distorted. In severe bilateral cases, the vowels become distorted and differentiation among physiologically similar vowels may be absent from the client's articulatory repertoire. Accurate consonant productions may be limited to a few phonemes, generally those with the greatest intensity (nasals, liquids, voiced plosives, etc.) and highest degree of visibility (bilabials, for example). Such clients will frequently evidence difficulty with correct voicing, pitch, intensity, and differential stress. The use of early amplification and speech therapy with such clients may significantly reduce the magnitude of the articulation disturbance.

In the case of bilateral deafness and in the absence of early therapeutic intervention, speech may be totally unintelligible. Articulatory attempts may be characterized by off-target vowel productions and unintelligible, highly distorted, consonantlike articulations. The client's habitual pitch level is typically inappropriate, and prosody is usually severely disturbed. In the case of fluctuating hearing loss, such as in cases of recurrent otitis media, the particular effect on articulation will depend on such variables as the frequency of the recurrence, the age span when affected and the magnitude of the episodic losses. Since these losses are typically conductive in nature, the client will generally evidence episodic mild to moderate hearing impairment. Some authorities maintain that such fluctuations in hearing sensitivity have a more deleterious affect on articulation development than a chronic loss of similar magnitude since they do not provide the child with an opportunity to compensate and adjust.

This type of hearing impairment may be far more common than realized by many clinicians. Middle ear infections are quite common in young children and an early recurrent pattern may well account for many of the articulation errors we see in children later diagnosed as having "functional" disorders. The prevalence of such losses is very high in cleft palate children. Early identification and medical treatment may obviate many of the problems associated with such losses.

Hearing losses may result from the following: outer ear conditions such as impacted wax, exostoses, congenital atresia; middle ear conditions such as tympanic membrane perforation, otitis media, cholesteatoma and otosclerosis; and, inner ear disturbances including noise exposure, Meniere's Disease, presbycusis, ototoxicity, and acoustic tumors. In light of the importance of normal hearing to articulation and considering the etiological significance of hearing loss, initial and routine audiological assessment of clients seen by the speech pathologist is probably warranted. Because of its potential importance and the special considerations involved, the final chapter is devoted to the topic of audiogenic articulation disorders.

Environmental Factors

So far we have discussed etiological factors that are inherent in the child. What of the child's environment? Are there factors external to the child or conditions that might contribute to or be directly causative of an articulation disorder? The answer would seem to be a tentative yes. Although I have indicated that only a modicum of stimulation would seem to be necessary for a child to develop normal articulation skills, there are family and environmental conditions that appear to functionally impede development.

Although one might not completely agree with Mowrer's Autism Theory of vocal development, there does seem to be some agreement that a child must, in some way, identify with his parents and have a relative sense of emotional security in order for articulation skills to develop on schedule. Emotional problems and insecurity during the critical speech-learning years may well interfere with a child's acquisition of a number of cognitive skills, including speech.

While there is no direct consistent evidence that articulation impaired youngsters are more emotionally unstable than their normal speaking peers, there does appear to be a higher incidence of coexisting problems having emotional overtones than one would expect by chance alone. For example, Van Riper and Irwin (1958), following a review of the subject, state that "we find infantile articulatory errors coinciding with other forms of infantile behavior, with thumb sucking, enuresis, temper tantrums, and whining — all in the same case."

Of course, these authors are referring to a special type of disorder known as "baby talk" or *infantile perseveration.* In such cases, as the name implies, articulation skills are characteristic of a child at a younger age of development and frequently characterized by a large number of /t/ and /d/ substitution errors. Such children may or may not show other forms of infantile behavior or maturational delay, although coexisting symptoms are not uncommon. It is not uncommon for a child who has a new baby brother or sister at home to adopt such an articulation pattern as an attention getting device. If articulation development has been within normal limits prior to some type of change in the family structure and if the infantile pattern is not a long-standing one, the likelihood is that it will prove self-correcting as the child begins to interact with peers in school, etc. Such acute onset problems are seldom sustained for long periods of time. However, this is quite different from the child who has never been on schedule in speech development.

There is some evidence to suggest that the parents of articulation impaired children tend to be slightly less well adjusted than other parents (Winitz, 1969; Powers, 1971). Andersland (1961) reports a correlation between articulation defectiveness and high maternal hostility and child rejection attitudes. Maternal personality is reported to be related but only at extreme levels. Such factors as parental neuroticism, ignorance of child raising practices, overly severe child discipline practices, poor social adjustment, history of divorce, etc., are frequently reported in the literature. Whether parental attitudes, such as hostility and rejection, are causally related to speech defectiveness or whether they emerge as a by-product of the child's speech deficit is unclear. However, it would appear that there is a higher incidence of parental maladjustment in cases where the child has an articulation defect.

Such attitudes as above, especially on the part of the mother, would certainly not be conducive to an emotionally stable environment and might well affect a child's overall development. Dickson (1962) reports that the mothers of children who retain their speech errors tend toward emotional immaturity and instability more than do mothers of children who spontaneously outgrow their articulation errors. This should not be interpreted as suggesting that a majority or even a large minority of the parents of articulation defective children are emotionally disturbed or socially maladjusted. It simply means that there is a higher incidence of such problems than one would expect in the general population and that the speech pathologist should be alert to the possible occurrence and disruptive influence of these factors on speech development.

Possibly related to the above, it has been demonstrated that the parents of articulation defective children have, on the average, achieved a lesser educational level and come from a lower socioeconomic strata than parents of nonimpaired children. As Templin (1957) demonstrates and as others confirm, the fathers' occupations tend to place them, as a group, in the lower socioeconomic range. This is reported to be especially true and significant for children in the four to seven-year-old age range. Winitz points out that educational and socioeconomic status may be macrovariables. The apparent relationship may reflect such variables as parental knowledge of child development, concern for speech, and the quantity and quality of speech and language stimulation and reinforcement found in the home.

As discussed previously, the role of imitation in the child's development of articulation skills is undoubtedly an important one. Thus, if the primary speech models in the child's home (the speech of parents and older brothers or sisters) are defective there is an increased likelihood that the child's speech will be similarly defective. Children frequently adopt the behaviors and mannerisms of those significant others in their environment. It is not uncommon for a parent to bring her child to the clinic and discover that she too has a problem or, in taking a case history, a clinician will frequently discover that the child's father has a similar speech defect.

According to Powers (1971), while there does not appear to be a correlation between sibling status in the family, when an older brother or sister has a defect there is an increased probability that the younger child will also manifest an articulation deficit. Of course, the probability is increased substantially in the case of twins. In some cases identical twins will develop deviate articulation patterns that are apparently intelligible to each other but not to others. In such cases of *twin ideoglossia* the dominant twin may or may not possess sufficient articulation skill to function as an interpreter for the brother or sister. In discussing the topic, Van Riper and Irwin (1958) state that the articulation errors of twins, both identical and fraternal, remain longer and that the problem "may in part be due to reciprocal imitation." The exact importance of good speech models in the child's environment and the role that imitation plays is still uncertain. However, it would appear to be of etiological significance in some clients.

Another factor that is probably important to the development of normal articulation skills is that of *need*. While the need to acquire basic speech and language ability is probably inherent in the child's biological and social being, the need for perfect articulation skills is probably contingent upon the degree of acceptance of the child's speech by those significant others in his environment. Parents typically learn their child's defective speech patterns and may respond appropriately to requests and communications whether or not such verbalizations are articulated correctly. It is not uncommon to have parents report that they can understand their child but that others, outside the family, cannot.

Total acceptance of their child's speech hardly provides motivation or need for improvement. By analogy, before one will learn to jump something must be put in the path. Why should a child attempt to produce a more difficult phoneme if a motorically easier one will suffice? As Van Riper and Irwin point out, many articulation errors frequently disappear during the child's first few years in school, probably because the environment is no longer unconditionally accepting his speech articulation. The importance of the developmental need factor is frequently stressed in parent conference sessions.

While a single environmental factor, if sufficiently severe, may precipitate an articulation disorder, multiple coexisting factors are more commonly to blame. In the majority of cases, I suspect that predisposing organic deficiencies (although subclinical in nature) may render the child susceptible to speech delay or articulation defect given certain negative environmental influences. Thus, environmental factors in most clients might be viewed as contributory rather than singularly causative.

ARTICULATION ERRORS

Throughout the text, reference has been made to various types of articulation errors and it is assumed that the reader has experienced little difficulty in comprehending the terminological referents in the general sense that they have been used. Now we will focus on specific types of errors with greater attention to definitional detail.

Consonants are misarticulated with far greater frequency than vowels. This is so much the case that many texts on articulation disorders and assessment do not include reference to specific vowel errors. Vowel errors, other than in cases of dialectal variation, suggest a more severe articulation impairment. To account for the greater frequency of occurrence of consonant errors we simply have to look at the physiological basis of consonant and vowel production. As discussed in Chapter 1, the syllable may well be the primary unit of speech production. Summarizing Stetson's 1951 work on motor phonetics, McDonald (1964) suggests that vowels function basically to shape the vocal tract for the syllable. As such, they require relatively gross articulatory posturing and are comparatively fixed or static in nature. Consonants, on the other hand, function to either release or arrest the syllable and, therefore, are more ballistic, require more rapid articulator movement and finer articulator adjustments and approximations. In this sense, they are motorically more complex than vowels and more difficult to produce accurately. Listeners are also more tolerant of slight variations in vowel productions than consonant articulations. It is therefore not surprising that children acquire and master vowel production prior to consonants and that vowels are more resistant to articulatory breakdown.

Specific Error Types

Consonant misarticulations may be categorized as errors of omission, substitution, distortion, or addition. While clients frequently manifest several types of articulation errors, a prevalent error type is typically noted. Of course this may vary in a given client with time dependent upon the relative stage of articulatory mastery. A number of authorities suggest that the prevalent type of articulation error is at least one index of the severity of an articulation disorder (Milisen, 1954; Irwin and Van Riper, 1958; Perkins, 1971). In descending order of severity, the articulation error types are as follows: (1) *omission,* in which the target phoneme is not produced and there is no substitution of a standard or nonstandard sound /ca/ for /cat/); (2) *substitution,* in which one standard phoneme is used in place of the target phoneme (/wed/ for /red/); (3) *distortion,* in which an off-target articulatory approximation of the target phoneme is produced resulting in an indistinct, nonstandard sound substitution (a lateral lisp for /s/); and, (4) *addition,* in which an inappropriate sound or syllable has been intruded into the articulatory sequence (/animamal/ for /animal/ or /buhring/ for /bring/).

Although we traditionally classify consonant articulation errors according to the guidelines above, it can be argued that all errors are generically substitutions. For example, distortion errors involve nonphonemic substitutions, i.e. the substitution of a nonstandard English sound for a target phoneme. Similarly, omission errors involve the substitution of a time gap in place of the target phoneme. The fact that a time gap or pause is present with omission errors suggests that the client is aware that something belongs in the space or temporal sequence.

The omission error is considered the most severe type of error since the substitution (time gap) least approximates the target phoneme. With substitution errors, the client obviously recognizes the need for a phoneme in the linguistic sequence but selects an incorrect one. The degree of approximation is closer than in the case of omissions. The particular severity of a given substitution error will depend upon the number of distinctive feature differences that exist between the phoneme substituted and the target phoneme. Thus, a /p/ for a /b/ substitution error would be considered less severe than a /t/ for a /b/. In the first case only the feature of voicing is in error while in the second both voicing and place of articulation (two feature errors) attributes are incorrectly applied. The /p/ approximates the /b/ to a greater extent than does the /t/.

In many cases of distortion errors, the client recognizes and appropriately selects the correct phoneme but does not achieve completely accurate phonetic realization. Typically, the production is an indistinct approximation of the target phoneme. As such, it approximates the target sound to a greater extent than either substitution or omission errors and is therefore considered less severe. The degree of approximation criterion of severity has been used by speech pathologists for many years. Van

Riper and Irwin (1958) suggest that children frequently go through stages of progressive approximation as a process of articulatory mastery, moving from omission to substitution, distortion, and, finally, correct articulation of a target sound.

However, there are exceptions to this general rule. For example, in cases where distortion errors are so gross that the intended target sound or even its phonemic class is unrecognizable the errors may be considered more severe than, say, simple sound substitutions with single distinctive feature errors. In addition, a prevalent error pattern characterized by distortion errors more probably reflects a phonetically based disorder with an organic etiology, such as cleft palate or dysarthria. Such cases are typically more resistant to speech therapy and, as such, might be considered more severe than cases in which the prevalent error pattern is characterized by phonemic substitutions.

Vowel errors are far less common than consonant misarticulations and, in general, are considered indicative of a more severe disorder. Their appearance is more common in cases of severe neuromotor impairment or hearing loss although they may also be prevalent in clients who have learned English as a second language (dialectal variations).

Vowels are described, in part, with reference to the location of the dorsum of the tongue in the oral cavity, e.g. high-low, front-mid-back, during the steady-state portion of production. Thus, the most common vowel errors are classified according to the malpositioning involved. Vowel misarticulations include the following: (1) *raising* errors, as in /pool/ for /pull/; (2) *lowering* errors, as in /sit/ for /seat/; (3) *fronting* errors such as /bat/ for /but/; and (4) *backing* errors, such as /sought/ for /sat/. Other vowel errors include *monothongization,* in which only one element of a diphthong is produced (a/aɪ) and *diphthongization,* in which a pure vowel is diphthongized. Additionally, vowel distortions may occur as the result of inaccurate lip rounding or the inappropriate use of stress. Vowel errors should be individually assessed using the principles of physiologic phonetics.

Articulation error type is only one factor in considering the nature and severity of a given disorder. Other factors such as error consistency, stimulability, and the frequency of occurrence of the error phoneme in the English language are of equal importance. Additional considerations such as a child's age and the number of sound errors are also taken into account in making clinical judgments. For instance, with very young children errors with the developmentally more advanced phonemes may be expected and are frequently considered age-appropriate. Of course, as previously discussed, these errors typically involve only single distinctive feature misapplications.

Error Consistency

A defective speech sound is seldom in error 100 percent of the time. A given error sound may be produced correctly by a client on some occasions or in certain phonetic contexts. This is to say that articulation errors are frequently inconsistent. Error inconsistency may reflect the influence of phonetic context and/or the degree to which a client has stabilized the sound in his phonetic repertoire. Traditional tests of articulation assess a client's ability to produce sounds in the initial, medial, and final positions of single words. The primary criticism of such testing practices is that it does not provide an adequate sample for the assessment of error consistency (McDonald, 1964). It is reasonable to assume, for example, that a client might be able to produce an /s/ sound with greater facility when it follows a /t/ sound than when it follows a /k/ sound. Thus McDonald argues convincingly that error sounds should be tested in a wide variety of phonetic contexts in order to determine error consistency and to discover possible "facilitating contexts" in which the sound is produced correctly or more nearly so. Such information may prove to be of value in clinical decision making.

Van Riper and Irwin (1958) suggest that sounds that have been stabilized and permanently learned are consistently produced. Thus, it might be reasonably argued that error sounds that are highly consistent have been stabilized as a part of the client's "ideolect" and are therefore more resistant to correction. High error consistency would therefore suggest a more severe defect. On the other hand, low error consistency (a high percentage of correct productions) might suggest that the client is in the process of acquiring or stabilizing the correct phoneme and, thus, may be indicative of a more favorable prognosis and a less severe problem. Inconsistency in the same phonetic context may suggest emergent phonemic development while inconsistency as a product of different phonetic contexts may be more indicative of a developmental phonetic generalization process. At any rate, error consistency has been demonstrated to be an important clinical consideration. Research suggests that children who are highly inconsistent in their error productions tend to outgrow their errors, with or without therapeutic intervention, while those who are highly consistent in their misarticulations are less likely to improve their speech without therapy (Sommers et al., 1967).

Error Stimulability

Stimulability refers to a client's ability to correctly produce or improve an error sound following stimulation by the clinician. Traditionally it is assessed by having the client attempt to imitate a clinician's auditory model of the target sound produced in isolation, in nonsense syllables, or in words. The degree or percentage (if multiple presentations are made) of improvement from spontaneous to imitative production is taken as the client's stimulability on the error sound in question.

Of course, many speech pathologists will go a step further in testing for stimulability if auditory modeling alone does not result in improvement. For example, a clinician may provide the client with brief phonetic instruction on the placement of the articulators for a given target sound and then again provide the auditory model. If the client is then able to correctly produce the sound, the clinician would note that the client is stimulable under the conditions of phonetic instruction and auditory modeling.

At any rate, error stimulability, assessed in the traditional manner, has been clinically and experimentally demonstrated to be a highly significant prognostic variable. Studies repeatedly demonstrate that spontaneous error sounds which are readily improved under imitative conditions are the easiest to correct with therapy but also have the greatest likelihood of proving to be self-correcting (Snow and Milisen, 1954; Carter and Buck, 1958; Farquhar, 1961; Sommers et al., 1967; Sommers, Cox, and West, 1972). As a general rule of thumb, those children who are highly stimulable on their error sounds have a higher probability of outgrowing their disorder spontaneously than children with low stimulability. All other variables equal, children in the latter group have the greatest need for therapy.

Articulation Index

Another index of the severity of an articulation disorder is the frequency of occurrence of a client's error sounds in the language. All phonemes do not have equal weight. Some occur with greater frequency than others. For example, the phonemes /t/, /n/, /r/, /s/, and /l/ occur with far greater frequency than /th/, /ch/, and /j/. Articulation errors on phonemes that occur with high frequency in the language will be more noticeable and reduce speech intelligibility to a greater extent than errors involving phonemes of low weight. This type of reasoning provided the impetus for Wood (1949) to develop an "Articulation Index" that weights each phoneme according to its frequency of occurrence in the language. Several articulation tests have been developed that allow a weighted score based on the Index. Such information is valuable in making clinical judgments of severity. It may also be of value in selecting the sound(s) with which to begin therapy. For example, given that two sounds are equally stimulable and all other considerations are equal, speech pathologists should probably begin working on the sound that occurs more frequently since correction will have the greater effect on improving speech intelligibility.

Thus, in summary, the variables of predominant error type, error consistency, stimulability, and phonemic weight, together with considerations such as the number of sounds in error and the young client's age, provide valuable clinical information concerning the severity of a disorder, the prognosis for improvement with or without therapy and, if indicated, with which sound(s) to begin therapy. These variables may also contribute information concerning the diagnosis of the articulation disorder type.

ARTICULATION DISORDER TYPES

As discussed in Chapter 3, articulation development involves at least two components. First, the developing child must acquire a conceptual awareness or knowledge of the sound system. He must establish a perceptual-cognitive image of those phonetic-acoustic variations in speech which signal phonemic difference (distinctive features) and must learn the language specific rules for combining these into phonemic segments. By analogy, he must learn the players and rules of the game. I have previously referred to this as phonemic development. Delayed or aberrant development (ideolect) in this respect will result in a *phonemically based* articulation disorder. In such cases, a specific distinctive feature or features have not been acquired by the client (absent from speech samples) or their attributes are misapplied (defective understanding of the rules of usage). Thus, a phonemically based articulation disorder reflects a deficit in the client's knowledge base.

In order for the developing child to fully participate in the communication act he must not only master a knowledge of the sound system but must also possess a speech mechanism and perceptual-motor system capable of mastering the complex motor coordinations required in speech production. In Chapter 3, I referred to this component of development as phonetic. Thus, articulatory production problems that are based on structural or neuroperceptual motor weakness or limitations are referred to as *phonetically based* disorders. Such disorders may be developmental in nature, resulting from neurological or structural limitations either present at birth or acquired during early childhood, or may be acquired after speech has been mastered as the result of injury, disease, stroke, etc.

Phonemic and phonetic development are interrelated and, to a certain extent, reciprocally facilitory. This is to say that they are not mutually exclusive, totally independent systems. They are, however, different components of the same system, and there seems to be little doubt that once a child has established a relative phonemic mastery there is still a need for a period of phonetic production practice and learning. However, it is the author's opinion that given relatively normal phonemic development, phonetic development will follow normally in the absence of structural or neurological involvement. Phonetic disorders may have obvious organic etiologies, as in cleft palate, severe tongue-tie, dysarthria, etc., or may result from less obvious causes such as developmental apraxia of speech as defined by Yoss and Darley (1974).

In recent years it has become increasingly popular to think of the majority of articulation disorders as phonemically based deficiencies involving the child's knowledge of the sound system. Winitz (1969) and others suggest that the majority of articulation errors may be traced to a lack of appropriate mastery of the phonemic component and that, for the most part, they are not problems of phonetic production. In supporting the position, these researchers point to the fact that very early in the child's development he is able to produce practically all sounds in the language, although not in meaningful contexts, i.e. purportedly he has the phonetic capability to produce the sounds, and that children are frequently able to correctly produce sounds that require roughly the same phonetic skills as their error sounds.

These observations, coupled with the advent of distinctive feature theory and clinical applications thereof, have convinced many speech pathologists that, in the absence of gross structural or neurological deficiencies, articulation disorders are predominantly phonemic deficits. However, it must be remembered that motor speech is an extremely complex process involving a sophisticated memory system that, when functioning normally, can store an extremely large number of articulatory targets and trajectories for sounds with an ability to make corrections according to contextual requirements.

The ability of a babbling child to produce a sound in a nonpurposive manner does not suggest a phonetic ability to produce the same sound in a purposive, contextual message. The latter is undoubtedly more complex and requires phonetic learning and memory programming. Further, just because a child has sufficient linguaalveolar facility to correctly produce the /n/ and /t/ sounds does not mean that he automatically has the phonetic skills required to produce the /s/ sound. Subtle neurological lesions involving the speech motor memory system may result in a phonetic "motor programming" disorder — apraxia of speech. Yoss and Darley's research suggests that developmental apraxia of speech (a phonetic disorder) may account for a significant percentage of the severe articulation disorders we see clinically. In such cases there is typically an absence of any readily obvious neurological impairment.

In phonemically based articulation disorders the predominant error pattern involves substitution errors. This is the case because the absence of a given feature attribute will result in a different phoneme being produced. Articulation errors are frequently inconsistent, depending upon the degree of error stabilization or the extent of feature generalization. Many of the sound errors may be accounted for on the basis of a single feature error. Clients with such disorders typically have difficulty with correct auditory discrimination of their error sounds, although they may be stimulable on some errors depending upon the degree of feature acquisition.

With phonetically based disorders, the typical error pattern is one of distortions and omissions. Error consistency is generally high, although, in cases of apraxia of speech in adults, the specific errors may be variable. Clients frequently are able to correctly discriminate between their errors and the correct

TABLE V

MAJOR DISTINCTIONS BETWEEN PHONETIC AND PHONEMIC
ARTICULATION DISORDERS

Phonemic Disorders	*Phonetic Disorders*
1. Predominantly substitution errors	1. Predominantly distortion and omission errors
2. Misarticulations related to specific feature errors	2. Misarticulations may be related to specific structural or neurologic deficit or motoric complexity
3. Errors may be inconsistent	3. Errors typically consistent
4. Difficulty with auditory discriminations of errors	4. Frequently normal ability to discriminate errors from target sounds
5. Client may be stimulable on some errors	5. Error stimulability is typically low
6. Structurally intact speech mechanism	6. Structural defect may be present
7. Diadochokinesis within normal limits	7. Diadochokinesis may be slow and labored
8. Oral sensation and perception normal	8. Oral astereognosis may be present

sounds although stimulability is typically low. Errors may reflect specific structural deficits or certain types of neurological impairments. Table V summarizes the major differences between phonetic and phonemic articulation errors.

Of course, phonetic and phonemic articulation errors may manifest themselves in the same client. The diagnostic picture is complicated by the fact that the deficits underlying phonetic mastery frequently also interfere with normal phonemic development. Although there are pure phonemic and phonetic disorders, the author's clinical experience suggests that in approximately 50 percent of the cases both phonetic and phonemic errors will be present. In such cases the author has typically used the prefix "predominantly" in designating the disorder type and has employed different treatment methods in working with the different error types. This will be discussed in the upcoming chapter on treatment.

REFERENCES

Achilles, R.: Communicative anomalies of individuals with cerebral palsy: I. Analysis of communicative processes in 151 cases of cerebral palsy. *Cerebral Palsy Rev, 16:*15-24, 1955.

Andersland, P.: Maternal and environmental factors related to success in speech improvement training. *J Speech Hear Res, 4:*70-90, 1961.

Bankson, N. and Byrne, M.: The relationship between missing teeth and selected consonant sounds. *J Speech Hear Disord, 27:*341-348, 1962.

Beasley, D., Shriner, T., Manning, W., and Beasley, D.: Auditory assembly of CVC's by children with normal and defective articulation. *J Commun Disord, 7:*127-133, 1974.

Carter, E. and Buck, M.: Prognostic testing for functional articulation disorders among children in the first grade. *J Speech Hear Disord, 23:*124-133, 1958.

Darley, F.: Appraisal of articulation. In Darley, F. and Spriestersbach, D.: *Diagnostic Methods in Speech Pathology.* New York, Har-Row, 1978.

Darley, F., Aronson, A., and Brown, J.: Differential diagnostic patterns of dysarthria. *J Speech Hear Res, 12:*246-269, 1969.

Darley, F., Aronson, A., and Brown, J.: *Motor Speech Disorders.* Philadelphia, Saunders, 1975.

Dickson, S.: Differences between children who spontaneously outgrow and children who retain functional articulation errors. *J Speech Hear Res,* 263-271, 1962.

Eisenson, J.: *Aphasia in Children.* New York, Har-Row, 1972.

Farquhar, M.: Prognostic value of imitative and auditory discrimination tests. *J Speech Hear Disord, 26:*342-347, 1961.

Fymbo, L.: The relation of malocclusion of the teeth to defects of speech. *Arch Speech, 1:*204-216, 1936.

Hardy, J. and Arkebauer, H.: Development of a test for velopharyngeal competence during speech. *Cleft Palate J, 3:*6-21, 1966.

Huber, N. and Kopp, A.: *The Practice of Speech Correction in the Medical Clinic.* Boston, Expression, 1942.

Johns, D. and Darley, F.: Phonemic variability in apraxia of speech. *J Speech Hear Res, 13:*556-583, 1970.

Kessler, H.: The relationship of dentistry to speech. *J Am Dent Assoc, 48:*44-49, 1954.

McDonald, E.: *Articulation Testing and Treatment: A Sensory-Motor Approach.* Pittsburgh, Stanwix, 1964.

McEnery, E. and Gaines, F.: Tongue-tie in infants and children. *J Pediatr, 28:*252-255, 1941.

Mecham, M., Berko, M., and Berko, F.: *Communication Training in Childhood Brain Damage.* Springfield, Thomas, 1966.

Milisen, R.: The disorders of articulation: a systematic clinical and experimental approach. *J Speech Hear Disord,* ASHA Monograph Supplement #4, 1954.

Perkins, W.: *Speech Pathology: An Applied Behavioral Science.* St. Louis, Mosby, 1971.

Powers, M.: Functional disorders of articulation: symptomatology and etiology. In Travis, L. (Ed.): *Handbook of Speech Pathology and Audiology.* New York, Appleton-Century-Croft, 1971.

Shankweiler, D. and Harris, K.: An experimental approach to the problems of articulation in aphasia. *Cortex, 2:*277-292, 1966.

Shriner, T., Holloway-Sayre, M., and Daniloff, R.: The relationship between articulatory deficits and syntax in speech defective children. *J Speech Hear Res, 12:*319-325, 1969.

Slorach, N. and Noehr, B.: Dichotic listening in stuttering and dyslalic children. *Cortex, 8:*224-232, 1972.

Snow, K.: Articulation proficiency in relation to certain dental abnormalities. *J Speech Hear Disord, 26:*209-212, 1961.

Snow, K. and Milisen, R.: The influence of oral versus pictorial representation upon articulation testing results. *J Speech Hear Disord,* Monograph Supplement #4, 29-36, 1954.

Sommers, R.: Factors related to the effectiveness of articulation therapy for kindergarten, first and second grade children. *J Speech Hear Res, 10:*428-437, 1967.

Sommers, R., Cox, S., and West, C.: Articulatory effectiveness, stimulability and children's performances on perceptual and motor tasks. *J Speech Hear Res, 15:*579-589, 1972.

Spriestersbach, D. and Powers, G.: Articulation skills, velopharyngeal closure and oral breath pressure of children with cleft palates. *J Speech Hear Res, 2:*318-325, 1959.

Spriestersbach, D. and Sherman, D.: *Cleft Palate and Communication.* New York, Acad Pr, 1968.

Subtelney, J. and Subtelney, J.: Intelligibility and associated physiological factors in cleft palate speakers. *J Speech Hear Res, 2:*353-360, 1959.

Templin, M.: Certain language skills in children, their development and inter-relationships. *Institute of Child Welfare Monograph Series,* No. 26. Minneapolis, U of Minn Pr, 1957.

Van Demark, D.: Misarticulations and listener judgments of the speech of the individuals with cleft palates. *Cleft Palate J, 3:*159-170, 1966.

Van Riper, C. and Irwin, J.: *Voice and Articulation.* Englewood Cliffs, P-H, 1958.

Wilson, F.: Efficacy of speech therapy with educable mentally retarded children. *J Speech Hear Res, 9:*423-433, 1966.

Winitz, H.: *Articulatory Acquisition and Behavior.* New York, Appleton-Century-Croft, 1969.

Yoss, K. and Darley, F.: Developmental apraxia of speech in children with defective articulation. *J Speech Hear Res, 17:*399-416, 1974.

CHAPTER 5

Assessment

E VALUATION OF ARTICULATION disorders is a multifaceted process and may involve both formal standardized test administration and informal assessment methods. The specific tests and assessment procedures selected for a given client will depend largely on the particular biases of the examiner, on the purpose(s) of testing and, in some instances, on the apparent etiology underlying the articulation defect. For example, the assessment procedures comprising a given test battery will probably vary depending upon whether the purpose is to identify the presence of a disorder (screening), to diagnose the specific nature of the disorder and classify the client in terms of developmental age equivalency, to obtain specific information relevant to prognosis and therapy planning, to determine the importance of a specific variable relative to the disorder, or to check on the progress made in therapy.

The test battery may also be altered in cases with known etiologies such as in cleft palate, neurologically based disorders or in the presence of severe hearing loss. This is done on the basis of a clinician's knowledge of some characteristically special problems frequently associated with such disorders. For instance, with a cleft palate client we may wish to include an articulation test that specifically samples the client's ability to produce phonemes with high intraoral breath pressure requirements. This, of course, would be based on our knowledge that such clients frequently misarticulate the phonemes requiring the impounding of air intraorally or the maintenance of sustained oral air pressure because of velopharyngeal insufficiency. Similarly, with neuromotor disorders special emphasis may be given to the assessment of the functional ability or motility of the speech mechanism during both speech and nonspeech activity. Thus, the specific tests selected and the particular procedures employed should be adapted to the information needs of the examiner.

In the final analysis, testing is simply a way of sampling a client's behavior and structuring clinical observations. Thus, whether a speech pathologist chooses to administer a standardized test or to structure his observations of the client's behaviors in a less formal manner, testing must be based on a firm understanding of the disorder in question and the behaviors of concern. The selection of a given test or assessment procedure should be based on the clinician's knowledge that the test in question will provide an efficient and valid method of sampling the behavior under consideration and that it will do so in a reliable manner.

During the early formative years of the profession, articulation skills were assessed by recording a sample of a client's connected speech and subjecting it to a phonetic analysis; such procedures are time-consuming and laborious. In order to reduce the amount of time involved in such testing and to increase assessment efficiency, members of the profession designed "articulation tests" that sample a client's ability to articulate the English phonemes in different positions of single words. For many years such testing practices were used and accepted as valid, i.e. they were felt to provide an adequate, representative sample of a client's articulation skills in spontaneous, connected speech.

While such "traditional" tests of articulation may provide useful information, it has become clear that they do not provide a representative sample of connected speech. As discussed in Chapter 1, we do not produce phonemes or words in an isolated, individual manner and articulatory accuracy may be greatly influenced by phonetic context and timing considerations. Thus, the production of a phoneme in the initial, medial, and final positions of three words can hardly be considered a valid sample. However, rather than return to the time-consuming practice of phonetically analyzing a connected speech sample, other tests that are considered to be more valid were developed. This will be discussed later in the chapter. At any rate, the moral of this little story is that we should give careful consideration to the selection of specific tests and assessment procedures. To reiterate, selection should be based upon our knowledge of the behavior we wish to sample and the validity (does it provide us with the information we are seeking) and reliability of the test.

It is important to remember that our clients are individuals and not pathologies. All too often I hear student clinicians refer to their "articulation cases" or their "cleft palate client" or their 10:30 appointment with their "aphasic patient." While diagnosis is important in identifying and classifying disorders and while diagnostic labels serve a communication function, they are all too often misused and may result in inappropriate management. It is important to identify the client's disorder type, however, it is equally important to recognize the fact that each client is an individual with variations in his presenting problem. If we treat all of our articulation cases with similar etiologies in the same manner we will undoubtedly mistreat many. Certainly, we should exercise caution in arriving at a diagnosis. Similarly, we should make certain that the diagnostic label, once applied, does not automatically dictate our therapy methods.

Along similar lines, we should avoid thinking about assessment in terms of a single "diagnostic" session preceding therapy. Obviously a preliminary assessment is needed in order to tentatively identify the disorder and plan therapy. However, in many cases additional assessment sessions are required and, even when sufficient information has been obtained to begin a therapy regimen, assessment should be an ongoing process. A good therapist is also a good diagnostician and should continuously assess the client's responses to specific approaches in order to determine therapeutic efficacy and to plan future intervention strategies. All too often our assessment focus stops once therapy is initiated. When this happens we are relegated to the status of a programmed teaching machine and the client suffers. Assessment should be an integral part of the therapy process and, as such, the concept of diagnostic therapy should be more widely adopted. In this sense, the best assessment tools are the ears, eyes, and mind of the clinician.

As suggested at the beginning of the chapter, the assessment of a client with an articulation disorder is a multifaceted process.

It typically includes the following: (1) the taking of a case history; (2) an oral peripheral examination; (3) the administration of a traditional diagnostic articulation test; (4) the administration of the Deep Test of Articulation to determine the consistency of identified errors and the influence of phonetic contexts; (5) a distinctive feature analysis to discern possible error patterns; (6) an assessment of error stimulability; and, (7) an assessment of speech sound discrimination ability. With such information it is usually possible to describe the nature, type, and severity of the disorder, to arrive at a reasonable prognosis, and to outline a tentative therapy plan.

THE CASE HISTORY

The importance of obtaining a good case history prior to testing cannot be overstated. Too frequently this aspect of assessment is treated in a perfunctory or cursory manner. It should not be. Invaluable information can be obtained through the combined use of preliminary questionnaires and the client or parent interview.

Preassessment session questionnaires are desirable in that they may provide exact structured information about the client from multiple sources simultaneously, i.e. questionnaires may be sent to the client or parents, the client's physician, teacher, or other professionals with knowledge about the client. They may also provide the clinician with questions he may wish to pursue in the interview session. There are several excellent reference sources that provide sample case history forms. One of the best is Darley and Spriestersbach's 1978 revised edition of *Diagnostic Methods in Speech Pathology.*

The interview provides an opportunity for the clinician to establish a positive working rapport with the client or parents and to obtain valuable client related information. It is probably best to conduct the interview in a comfortable relaxed setting and to interact with the informant using a conversational mode. While notes may and probably should be taken, it is usually unwise to complete a questionnaire during the interview. It tends to result in an overly formal atmosphere and may restrict the information flow from the informant. The speech pathologist should explain the purpose of the interview and should then ask questions in a nondirective manner, allowing the informant to do most of the talking.

Questioning should be primarily for the purpose of focusing the informant's attention on areas of concern. While some "yes or no" type questions may be called for, they should be kept to a minimum. In addition to obtaining specific, factual information, the interview provides an opportunity to obtain valuable insight into the perceptions of the client or parents regarding the magnitude of the "problem." It also provides the clinician with a chance to do some preliminary "speech hygiene" type counseling and to answer some of the questions and concerns of the client or family members.

Whether obtained through questionnaires or the interview format, initial intake information should include a description of the presenting problem, a history of the speech disorder, a medical history, a developmental history, a familial history, a review of any previous counseling or treatment for the disorder, and an identification of any other potentially predisposing, precipitating, or maintaining variables that might be important in arriving at a diagnosis, prognosis, or therapy plan.

Once the purpose of the intake interview has been discussed with the informant it is probably best to begin with a request for a *description of the problem*. In all likelihood the client has been referred for help by someone who has perceived a problem. The emphasis here is on the word *perceived*. What one person perceives as a serious problem another may regard as a minor deviation. In this respect it should be noted that while the speech pathologist can describe the number and type of misarticulations present in a given client, only the client and his immediate family can describe the magnitude of the problem. Thus, it is important to arrive at an estimate of the magnitude of the perceived problem. This can best be obtained by having the informant describe the problem in his own words. The manner in which it is characterized may provide valuable insights for the clinician concerning client and parental attitudes. Such information may be useful to the clinician when later considering possible problems with motivation, home carry-over activity, or when considering the possibility of a parent-directed therapy approach with certain young clients.

In addition to specific characterizations of the speech defect, the clinician should elicit information concerning how well family members understand the client, whether or not those outside of the immediate family are able to understand him, the method(s) by which the client communicates his needs and wants to others (oral-verbally, gesturally, or through a combination of the two), and the degree to which the speech defect may be affecting the client's social, emotional, or, if applicable, academic growth. Of course, some of this should be pursued more fully in taking a developmental history.

Related to the description of the problem, the clinician should inquire about the *history of the speech defect.* Specific information concerning the onset and progression of the problem should be elicited. Questions relating to the age the problem was first noticed, who first became concerned about the client's speech, the circumstances surrounding the onset of the problem, and whether or not the problem has become worse or lessened over time should be asked. It is important to determine whether the articulation problem was present and apparent when the child first began attempting speech or at an age when most children begin talking or whether onset occurred later in the child's speech developing years. If the latter is the case, the exact circumstances surrounding the onset should be explored fully. Information concerning any attempts to treat the problem, by parents or other professionals, should be obtained. The nature of such treatment and the results, if any, should be recorded for later reference.

A *medical history* should be taken. While much of this can be obtained in preassessment questionnaires, it is probably best to pursue the subject in the interview. Parents do not always understand the relationships between certain medical conditions and speech development and may, therefore, omit some potentially valuable information from a questionnaire.

Information concerning the birth history should be obtained. Questions concerning possible complications during pregnancy (maternal rubella, trauma, illness, etc.), the length of gestation (was the child born prematurely), the length and difficulty of labor, the manner of delivery (normal or caesarian), and complications during or immediately post delivery (forceps injury, premature separation of the placenta, problems with spontaneous respiration, circulation, jaundice, etc.) should be asked.

The speech pathologist should also obtain information relevant to the medical history during infancy and childhood. Much of this may be obtained from the child's pediatrician or family physician either on the phone or through a medical questionnaire. The interview might be used to obtain expansion or clarification of the information. Regardless of the method, however, information concerning unusual childhood diseases, protracted fevers, hospitalization record, falls (relevant to possible head injury), chronic colds or upper respiratory problems, allergies, earaches or infections, problems with tonsils and adenoids, and past or present medical treatment (including medications) regimens should be obtained.

Of course, any one of the above areas, if applicable, might be explored in depth. For example, if a parent reported that a child had experienced a bad fall with a blow to the head at an earlier age, the clinician would certainly want to pursue the matter by asking questions: did he lose consciousness; was he hospitalized; did it cause a concussion or result in a skull fracture or penetration; was there any nausea or vomiting afterwards; was he drowsy or did he seem disoriented and confused afterwards; did he experience any blurring of vision; etc.

Medical history information can be extremely important to the speech pathologist and can be supportive of test information obtained later in the assessment. It may provide information on a previously existing condition (no longer present) that might have bearing on the etiology, diagnosis, prognosis, or therapy plan. The speech pathologist will also want to ask the informant if the client's physician is aware of a speech problem and, if so, in what manner he might have counseled the parents or family. This may provide insight relative to the amount and nature of information the client or parents have and may provide a springboard for some preliminary counseling. Nation and Aram

(1977) provide an excellent reference on the specifics of taking a medical history.

A *developmental history* should be taken. Information concerning a client's overall speech, physical, emotional, and social development may provide data supportive of a specific etiology or may suggest the extent to which the articulation defect is an integral part of a general developmental maturational delay. Tables listing the sequences and average ages of landmark language, motor, and social development may be found in an excellent reference text by Nicolosi, Harryman, and Kresheck (1978) entitled *Terminology of Communication Disorders*. The approximate ages at which a child attained important developmental milestones should be recorded. While parents may be able to recall the major milestones, they are frequently unable to remember many. The clinician may be able to elicit approximate ages by verbally assisting parents in reconstructing various activities that the child may have engaged in at different ages. Of course, the reliability of parental memory, especially in families with many children, may be questionable. Some of the information may be obtained from pediatrician's records or, if available, from a "baby book."

At any rate, minimal information should include such examples as the approximate ages at which a child first sat unsupported, crawled, stood with assistance, took his first independent steps, was weaned from a bottle, fed himself with a spoon, stood on one foot, was able to jump and skip, etc., began imitating the sounds of others during babbling, said his first meaningful word, used his first holophrastic sentence, began using two and three word sentences routinely, began responding appropriately to his name and "yes or no," began understanding short, simple commands, two level commands, etc., was able to identify the basic parts of the body, began to understand prepositions and concepts of size, color, and number; began imaginary independent play, began playing with other children in an interactive manner, was bowel and bladder trained during the day, was able to sleep through the night without soiling, and began to explore the world around him independent of his parents. Of course, these are intended only as examples of the type of information important in a child's developmental history. The examiner will want to obtain more specific data where possible and will certainly wish to explore problem areas in the child's overall development.

Questions concerning developmental progression or the abrupt disruption in some aspect of the child's development should be asked. It is quite appropriate to ask parents if they feel their child is generally happy, emotionally secure, and well-adjusted and to make inquiry into possible problems concerning parent-child dependency, interaction with siblings, peers, etc. Parents frequently have insights concerning their child's development that can be useful to the clinician in understanding the client and that cannot be obtained in the course of a one or two hour testing session. An honest, open, and concerned attitude on the part of the clinician, coupled with the appropriate questions, may elicit the information needed.

Either as part of the developmental history or as a separate section, if applicable, information concerning a client's *academic record* in school should be obtained. A child's performance during the elementary school grades can provide valuable information. Undoubtedly, a child's placement in a special education class or in a class for children with specific learning disabilities may provide valuable background information relevant to a given client's ability to process and code symbolic information. In such cases, the clinician should seek specific information concerning the child's individual learning problems. Children with moderate and severe articulation defects frequently also have difficulty in learning to read and with the language arts in general. They may also have difficulty with arithmetic concepts since it involves an abstract symbol system.

It should be mentioned that speech is typically the primary symbol system through which other systems (reading, writing, arithmetic) are acquired, e.g. written letters (graphemes) are recoded in terms of the sounds of speech (phonemes) as they are initially learned. Difficulty with the phonemic system will, in many cases, cause problems for the child in learning secondary symbol systems. While this is somewhat of a generalization, it appears to be true in many cases and may explain the frequent relationship observed between articulation impairment and poor academic performance. Information obtained from teachers, school psychologists, remedial reading specialists, etc., can be highly useful to the speech pathologist in arriving at a diagnosis and planning a program of therapy.

A positive *family history* of speech and language impairment may be significant. While this is especially true with members of the immediate family, it may also be important when noted in more distant relatives as well. It is well known that a child may imitate the defective speech patterns of a mother, father, or older brothers and sisters. However, even when the influence is not immediate, a positive history may suggest a genetic or familial predisposition to articulatory difficulty. Such information may prove useful when considering etology, familial attitudes, and in planning counseling and therapy strategies.

It is probably best to close the intake interview by asking the informant if there is anything else, not covered, that might help you better understand the client or if there are any questions concerning the topics discussed. It may also provide an opportunity to explore some points made previously during the interview that might not have been appropriately pursued at the time. Questions may be asked to obtain clarification of previously given information or as a reliability check on the informant's memory.

If not previously addressed, information concerning a client's home environment might be pursued. For example, were there any family problems that might have caused an unstable home environment during the child's critical speech learning years? Does the child have ample opportunity to interact with children his own age at his present home location? Information of this type should certainly be obtained at some point during the interview. It must be remembered that an articulation defect is symptomatic of some underlying cause, be it a single etiology or multiple in nature. A good case history exploration may reveal the underlying culprit(s).

THE ORAL PERIPHERAL EXAMINATION

The first step in the direct examination of a client with a reported articulation defect is to assess the structural and functional adequacy of the speech mechanism and supporting structures. The purpose of the examination is to: (1) Identify any structural defects which, singly or in combination with other problems, may have caused or contributed to an articulation disorder. (2) Assess the mobility of the articulators with reference to the range of motion and rate of movement needed for normal speech production. (3) Detect any associated defects or dysfunctions involving phonation, respiration and resonance. A thorough examination requires that the clinician have a detailed knowledge of the anatomy and physiology of the speech mechanism. An excellent reference source is Bateman's *A Clinical Approach to Speech Anatomy and Physiology* (Thomas, 1977).

In addition to knowledge, it is important that the clinician have experience in examining the mechanism. Unlike standardized objective tests, the oral peripheral examination primarily involves observations by the clinician and requires a judgment of normal or deviant and the degree to which deviant structures may impede speech production or development. In the final analysis, the speech pathologist is interested in the functional adequacy of the mechanism relative to speech production requirements. However, he must also subjectively assess structural adequacy in order to determine the possible etiology underlying the functional impairment. In this respect, it is important for the examiner to decide whether or not speech improvement is possible in light of a given structural defect and, if not, to consider appropriate referral for physical management. The best tools that the clinician can bring to bear on the examination are a firm knowledge of the anatomy, an understanding of physiological phonetics, and experience in examination.

It is important to remember that all people are not equally susceptible to a given defect even when the magnitude of the defects are identical. People evidence differential abilities to compensate. However, as a general rule of thumb a child will not be able to compensate for structural deformity if a single defect is very large or if there are multiple deviations. It is therefore important to note all deviations from normal for later consideration, even though a single deformation may not be considered a potentially significant causative agent. Darley and Spriestersbach (1978) suggest the use of a four point scale in rating the adequacy of the structures. The suggested scale involves rating the structures as follows: (1) *Normal;* (2) *Slight Deviation* — probably no adverse effect on speech; (3) *Moderate Deviation* — possible adverse effect on speech, remedial services may be required, particularly if other structures of the speech mechanism are also involved; and (4) *Extreme Deviation* — sufficient to prevent normal production of speech, modification of structure is required, either with or without clinical speech services.

For structural modification, referral is typically made to a plastic surgeon, when the defect involves palatal or maxillofacial deformities, or to a dentist or orthodontist, when the defect involves the teeth. Of course, the decision to attempt structural modification through surgery or orthodontia rests with the surgeon or orthodontist. However, the speech pathologist should work with these professionals and may rightfully point out the relationship between a certain structural defect and the impaired speech physiology. To attempt therapy in the face of a defect that severely limits the prognosis may be harmful and frustrating for both the client and clinician. In questionable or borderline cases the best practice is usually to enroll the client in a trial therapy regimen and to refer to the appropriate specialist for consultation.

Below is an outline discussion covering the various aspects of the examination. Although the various structures are discussed separately, it should be understood that speech production is a synergistic process involving an overlapping interaction among all of the structures.

General Observations

Observations concerning the overall structural adequacy and integrity of the central and peripheral nervous system may begin at the time when the speech pathologist first meets the client. The clinician may observe the client's general body posture, his ability to maintain head balance while seated, and his gait pattern on the way to the examination room. Problems in maintaining an erect head posture or balance, or an awkward or deviant walking pattern may be indicative of neurological involvement and may suggest the need of more detailed examination. Specific note should be made of any involuntary movement (tremor) of the extremities or facial area.

The general configuration and state of the facial musculature should be observed. Notation should be made of any facial asymmetry, structural or positional deviation of the mandible, left or right deviation of the nasal septum, drooping of the face (including the eyelid) on one side or the other, greater retraction of one corner of the mouth than the other, and any scarring of the lip or other facial areas (unilateral or bilateral). Scarring of the upper lip on one side or bilaterally may be due to a congenital cleft lip and may be associated with a cleft of the palate as well. Facial drooping or marked asymmetry, together with possible drooling and swallowing difficulty (dysphagia) is frequently the result of neurological impairment and should certainly be noted.

Additional observations should be made of the lips, nose, and anterior mouth areas. In addition to scarring, the clinician should make note of any asymmetry of the lips. Do the lips appear to be of sufficient mass? Is the upper lip short or does it seem to be unusually tight or restricted in movement capability? Do the lips touch at rest? Can the client produce the bilabial phonemes? Asymmetry of the nose may signify the presence of a congenital defect. In addition to deviations of the nasal septum, notice should be taken of the symmetry of the alar wings. Is there any unusual depression or flaring of the alar wings? Normally during passive respiration the mouth is closed. Are there any signs of mouth breathing? Is the mouth held open with the tongue protruded slightly during quiet breathing? This may signal problems with excessive adenoid tissue or other forms of partial obstruction of the nasopharyngeal air way.

The speech pathologist should also make note of the client's general respiratory pattern. Normally during quiet respiration observable movement is restricted to the abdomen and mid-thoracic regions of the body. The normal breathing rate is approximately fifteen to twenty inhalation-exhalation cycles per minute. The clinician should note irregularities in the breathing pattern, such as elevation of the clavicles during inhalation or a rapid shallow breathing rate. Record should also be made of any audible sound during normally quiet respiration.

The Lips

As is the case in examining all of the articulators, our primary concern relates to their physiological adequacy with reference to speech production. Due to the mobility of the lower lip, structural deviations involving the upper lip alone are seldom of sufficient magnitude to interfere with normal production of the bilabial phonemes. However, neurological disorders may render the lips paretic and imprecise or off-target bilabial articulations may result.

This is equally true for both the bilabial consonants as well as for the vowels that require lip rounding or retraction. Thus, it is important to check labial mobility in addition to the structural observations suggested above. The speech pathologist should ask the client to protrude and retract the lips as quickly as possible, demonstrating the action. Range of movement should be noted, as well as any apparent difficulty in accomplishing the task. The normal individual should be able to protrude (purse) and retract the lips two times per second. The clinician may then have the client produce the vowels (u) and (æ) alternately to observe the same process during speech production. The client may then be asked to open and close the lips rapidly. Repetition of the syllable (pʌ) may be used for this purpose. The normal individual should be able to produce the syllable four or five times per second. The clinician might also observe for the adequacy of the labial seal relative to the client's potential to produce the bilabial plosives.

The Tongue

The tongue is the most important oral articulator concerned with the production of speech sounds. It is normally capable of rapid fine motor movement and, in coordination with the other articulators, has primary responsibility in modifying the size and shape of the oral cavity. Disturbances of the structure or functional mobility of the tongue may have a marked deleterious effect on speech articulation.

Congenital defects in lingual structure include midline clefts, malformation, and asymmetry, inappropriate size in relation to the dental arches (*microglossia, macroglossia*), partial or complete absence of tongue formation and a short and extended lingual frenum. The author's clinical experience suggests, however, that with the exception of the last category, these problems are rather rare. When defects in the formation or size of the tongue do occur they are typically obvious and may be directly visualized and described by the speech pathologist. There are no available objective indices and their identification and definition is made on the basis of subjective assessment and description. The speech pathologist should make every effort to determine the potential impact of such deformations on speech development and production capability.

Examination should be done both with the tongue at rest (inside the oral cavity) and then with the tongue protruded. The examiner will need a good light source and a tongue blade is frequently useful. Examination of the tongue at rest may be accomplished by lowering the client's mandible. The examiner should do this since asking the client to open his mouth frequently results in automatic tensing or protrusion of the tongue. With the mouth open, the tongue may be examined. Is tongue carriage normal? Does it appear to rest more forward in the mouth than normal? Does the size of the tongue appear to be appropriate relative to the size and circumference of the dental arches and the anterior-posterior dimensions of the oral cavity? Does the tongue appear to be normally formed and symmetrical?

In adult clients, the partial or complete absence of the tongue (aglossia) is far more commonly the result of surgery to remove oral cancer than congenital deformation. Similarly, lingual asymmetry is more commonly the result of long standing paretic conditions. Long standing unilateral flaccid paralysis involving the cranial nerves may result in tissue wastage and atrophy on the affected side. The affected side of the tongue may appear shriveled and small in comparison to the unaffected side. Such a condition may appear alone or in combination with other signs of weakness of the head, neck, and facial musculature on the same side. Such symptoms are diagnostic of unilateral brain stem damage or direct cranial nerve lesions. The interested reader is referred to Chapter V of Darley, Aronson, and Brown's text, *Motor Speech Disorders* (1975).

The *lingual frenum* should be routinely examined. An overly extended and short frenum may severely restrict tongue mobility. In severe cases, the client may not be able to raise the tip of the tongue above the level of the lower incisors. The frenum may be seen to extend to the tip with an indentation in the midline of the tongue tip. With the tongue completely anchored to the floor of the mouth, the examiner will not be able to raise the tip with a tongue blade. However, visualization of the frenum is usually possible by elevating the sides of the tongue near the region of the lingual apex.

Most cases will not be so severe and will call for a judgment from the speech pathologist with reference to the potential negative affect on speech production. The range of tongue movement should be examined in this respect. Can the client protrude the tongue interdentally to a sufficient degree to produce the /th/ phoneme? Can the client raise the tongue tip or apex sufficiently to achieve correct articulation of the /s/, /z/, /t/, /d/, /l/, and /n/ phonemes? If the client has compensated for his lack of anterior tongue mobility, are his adaptations maladaptive and have they resulted in a coarticulation problem affecting other phonemes? These are considerations that the speech pathologist should make in deciding whether or not to refer the client for possible clipping of the frenum. While the speech pathologist should be cautious in arriving at such a decision, he should not hesitate if it is obvious that the condition is significantly interfering with a client's speech development and production ability.

Range, speed, and accuracy of tongue movement should be checked in both speech and nonspeech activity. The examiner should have the client protrude, lateralize, depress, and elevate the tongue, noting any difficulty or awkwardness. For some clients, demonstration of the desired behavior by the examiner will be necessary. In case of *neurological impairment,* the client's attempts may be slow, labored, and awkward and range of motion may be limited. In cases of severe paralysis the client may not be able to perform the tasks at all. However, obvious head, neck, and facial weakness are typically present in such clients. In cases of paresis, the tongue will normally deviate to the affected side upon attempts at protrusion. Lingual or facial tremor may be present in some clients.

Difficulty in tongue movement in the absence of any discernible paralysis, weakness, or incoordination may suggest the presence of an *oral apraxia.* Such clients have difficulty with purposive planned oral movements but may demonstrate completely normal ability when carrying out the activity on an automatic level. For example, when asked to protrude their tongue they may have great difficulty but, later in the examination, the clinician may observe them licking their lips automatically. Similarly, when asked to pretend that they are blowing out a match, great difficulty may be encountered but the client may be able to blow out a real match without hesitation or effort. Such a condition may coexist with *apraxia of speech,* an articulation disorder to be discussed in some depth later in the book.

Any slowness, awkwardness, or limited range of motion in protruding the tongue, moving it from side to side or up and down or licking the lips should be noted. Additionally, the examiner should check the client's ability to curl the tongue up and back, to touch the alveolar ridge with the tongue tip and to touch the soft palate with the dorsum of the tongue. The speech pathologist can have the client produce the monosyllables /tʌ/ and /kʌ/ and the bisyllable /tʌkʌ/ as rapidly as possible to check the speed of tongue movement. Normally, a client should be able to produce the monosyllables at a rate of four or five per second and at least three bisyllable productions per second. The ability to start and stop movement of the articulators is referred to as *diadochokinesis* and will be discussed later in this section.

The Teeth

As per the discussion in Chapter 4, the teeth contribute significantly to our ability to correctly articulate the labiodental, linguadental, and linguaalveolar fricatives. Thus, significant deviations in the alignment of individual teeth or relationship between the upper and lower teeth may contribute to an articulation defect. Missing teeth or the presence of a dental appliance or oral prosthesis may also interfere with an individual's ability to correctly articulate speech sounds.

Few speech pathologists hold degrees in dental science and, therefore, cannot and should not make diagnoses concerning the dental health of a client. However, as part of the oral peripheral examination they should examine the teeth and make note of any deviations that might interfere with normal speech production. For example, the front teeth provide a cutting edge for the sharp clear production of /s/ and /z/. Thus, missing front teeth may result in a distorted production of these phonemes. Similarly, the lateral teeth assist us in allowing the air stream to be directed down the midline of the mouth. Missing lateral teeth may result in a lateralization of the air stream, frequently observed in clients with lateral lisps.

The examiner should also note the alignment of the teeth. With normal occlusion the individual teeth are well aligned and the upper and lower dental arches have a normal front to back and side to side relationship. Although there is a good deal of variation in what can be considered "normal," in general, the upper dental arch is somewhat larger than the lower, the upper first molars are placed approximately one half of a tooth forward relative to the lower and the upper front teeth rest slightly forward and marginally overlap the lower. Any significant deviations relative to missing teeth, individually malaligned teeth, or malocclusion should be noted. For visualization of the various types of malocclusions discussed in Chapter 4 and for additional information, such as the schedule for eruption of the deciduous and permanent teeth, the reader is referred to texts by Bateman (1977) and Shafer, Hine, and Levy (1974).

Ill-fitting orthodontic appliances or loose dentures may interfere with normal articulation. Most children fitted with braces or adults fitted with dentures are able to adapt to their new structures in a short period of time and the early misarticulations (usually slight distortions) prove self-correcting within a few days or, at most, within a few weeks. However, in the presence of other defects, such adaptation may not occur and speech therapy may be needed. The author has also experienced geriatric clients who have articulation difficulty secondary to loose or ill-fitting dentures. As an individual grows older the dental arches may grow smaller. Thus, dentures that once fit properly become loose and interfere with normal articulation. If the client also suffers a dysarthria, poorly fitting dentures may further reduce speech intelligibility. In such cases, dental referral is obviously indicated. In addition to braces and dentures, other oral prostheses, such as maxillary expanders, obturators and palatal lift prostheses may, in some cases, interfere with normal articulation. In such cases the speech pathologist should consult with the dentist, orthodontist, or prosthodontist concerning the planned length of time that the prosthesis is to be in place, its fit, and its effect on speech.

The Palate

Examination of the hard and soft palate is done by observation with the aid of an adequate light source. Defects in structural adequacy are typically visible. The primary purpose of the palate is to provide separation between the oral and nasal cavities. Such separation is necessary for the generation of intraoral air pressure associated with the production of most phonemes, especially the plosives, fricatives, and affricates.

Clefts or openings in the palate, if large enough to be visible upon inspection, will allow air to escape through the nasal cavity and may adversely affect the correct production of these phonemes. Clefts may occur at any location along the lines of palatal fusion. Clefts may be midline only, involving varying degrees of the hard and soft palate; they may extend through the alveolus on either or both sides; or they may involve only the soft palate or only the alveolus. Surgically unrepaired clefts should be described in terms of the location (portions of the palate involved) and size (width) of the cleft.

In this day and time it is somewhat unusual to examine an older child with a totally unrepaired palatal cleft. However, it is not unusual to find clients in which a portion of the palate has been intentionally left unrepaired by the plastic surgeon for one reason or another. In such cases, the speech pathologist should describe the unsutured cleft and should make inquiry concerning the surgeon's plans for future correction of the defect.

It is also not uncommon to find palatal openings (not complete clefts) in the palate in clients who have undergone palatal closure operations. Such openings are called *fistulas* and typically result from a failure of the palate to heal properly following suturing or a tearing apart of the palatal shelves along the suture line. Fistulas may occur at any location. Darley and Spriestersbach (1978) state that "a fistula in the anterior and middle thirds of the palate is likely to result in greater escape of air pressure in speech than one at either the extreme anterior or posterior margin of the palate." As with palatal clefts, fistulas should be carefully described and their potential impact on the client's ability to generate intraoral air pressure for speech assessed.

In addition to the integrity of the palate, the speech pathologist should make note of the size and shape of the palatal vault. The size and shape of the palatal vault largely dictate the size of the oral cavity and the amount of space for lingual movement. An excessively narrow vault with either an extremely high or unusually flat contour (arch) may restrict tongue movement to the degree that normal linguapalatal articulations may be difficult. In such cases, although admittedly rare, maladaptive posturing and articulatory compensations may be manifest.

The soft palate (velum) serves as an articulator. During the production of oral phonemes the velum normally moves up and back, making contact with the pharynx in order to seal off the nasal port and allow separation between the oral and nasal cavities. The failure of the velum to make contact with the pharynx will result in air pressure being directed through the nose and an inability to generate sufficient intraoral air pressure for correct articulation. Thus, it is important to examine the adequacy of the *velopharyngeal mechanism*.

The structural integrity of the velum should first be examined. Although the velum may not be cleft, it may be congenitally short, to the extent that contact with the pharynx is not possible even with good up and back movement. The velum may also be heavily scarred as the result of surgery to close a cleft. In such clients, the scar tissue may function to restrict movement and interfere with the velum to pharynx excursion. These problems should be noted.

Velar movement may be observed directly by having the client repeatedly produce the /a/ sound. While the amount of superior-posterior movement of the velum can be visualized in such a manner, actual velopharyngeal contact cannot. In cases of marked velopharyngeal insufficiency the lack of movement or contact may be obvious from direct inspection. However, in borderline cases where significant movement is occurring but the examiner is uncertain about velopharyngeal closure, other methods of assessment should be employed.

For speech pathologists working in medical settings, lateral x rays (stills or cinefluorograms) may be made of the velopharyngeal region with the client at rest and during phonation and speech activity. Inspection of the x rays allows for assessment by providing a direct, lateral visualization of the velopharyngeal mechanism.

Direct visualization of the mechanism is also possible through endoscopy. Taub (1966) designed an endoscope expressly for this purpose. The Taub Oral Panendoscope is a tubular device with a viewer at one end and a mirror and light source at the other. By introducing the mirror end into the oropharynx, visualization of the nasopharynx and velopharyngeal movement is possible. Some experience with the instrument is necessary.

Many speech pathologists do not have access to x-ray facilities or endoscopic equipment and must rely on indirect methods of assessing velopharyngeal sufficiency. Indirect procedures include oral manometry, the Puff-Cheek Test, and articulation testing.

Oral manometry involves having the client blow into a manometer, which registers the amount of air pressure generated through the mouth. The typical procedure is to ask the client to blow into the manometer three times with the nares open and three times with the nares occluded (pinched together by the examiner). The highest reading obtained with the nares unoccluded is placed over the highest reading obtained with the nares occluded to form a manometric "competency" ratio. The extent to which the pinching of the nares is required to provide a nasal seal reflects the degree to which the velopharyngeal mechanism is inadequate. (It is interesting to note that in this respect children with velopharyngeal inadequacy frequently manifest nares constriction during attempts to produce the pressure phonemes.)

The resultant ratio, in cases of complete velopharyngeal adequacy, should be one. The smaller the resultant ratio (fraction) the less competent the mechanism. Ratios above .89 infer velopharyngeal sufficiency, ratios from .50 to .89 suggest inconsistent or marginal sufficiency and ratios below .49 are interpreted as reflecting a completely inadequate mechanism (Johnson, 1974; Powers, 1962; Spriestersbach, Moll, and Morris, 1961; and Van Demark, 1966). While manometric ratios have been shown to be only moderately correlated with speech defectiveness, they may serve as an index of gross velopharyngeal adequacy.

The Puff-Cheek Test (Fox and Johns, 1970), as the name implies, involves having the client puff out his cheeks. Several demonstrations by the examiner may be necessary. The examiner then applies pressure medially (squeezes the client's cheeks) and notes whether the impounded air pressure releases through the lips (labial release) or the nose (velar release). The individual with adequate velopharyngeal closure will evidence a labial release. In the case of an inadequate mechanism, the client will either not be able to puff out his cheeks at all or with the application of medial pressure the marginally sufficient velopharyngeal contact will break down and the impounded air will release through the nose. As a check on the validity of the procedure, the client's ability to puff out his cheeks with the tongue protruded and held outside the mouth is checked. A client's ability to generate and impound intraoral air pressure under this condition precludes the possibility that the client was using a compensatory linguavelar contact to achieve success on the first test. As with manometry, the Puff-Cheek Test is an indirect method and cannot be used in the case of a cleft or fistula in the hard palate. In such cases, the air would escape nasally regardless of the adequacy of the velopharyngeal mechanism.

The single best indirect procedure for assessing nasopharyngeal closure is articulation testing using high breath pressure phonemes, i.e. plosives, fricatives, and affricates. In a 1974 study, the author demonstrated high correlations between the results of articulation testing using plosives and fricatives, x-ray data (cinefluorograms) and endoscopic test findings.

Clients with less than 50 percent correct production of these phonemes revealed velopharyngeal inadequacy on x-ray and endoscopic examination. Those with over 90 percent correct production scores demonstrated adequate velopharyngeal closure. Thus, for those without access to x-ray facilities or endoscopic equipment, the test battery should include the following, in order of priority: (1) direct visual examination of velar movement; (2) articulation testing with plosives, fricatives, and affricates; (3) the Puff-Cheek Test; and, (4) oral manometry.

The Fauces

The fauces or faucial isthmus is simply the opening between the oral cavity and oropharyngeal region. It is bounded superiorly by the soft palate, inferiorly by the tongue, and laterally by the faucial pillars. It is easily visualized upon direct oral examination. Excluding problems with the palate or tongue, the primary structures or tissue of concern are the faucial tonsils and anterior and posterior faucial pillars or folds. The concern arises over the patency of the isthmus. In cases of extremely large and medially distended faucial tonsils, the oral air way may be partially occluded resulting in poor oral resonance. It is also possible that extremely large faucial tonsils may so distort the pillars (palatoglossus and palatopharyngeus muscles) that normal muscular function is disturbed. This may be especially critical for the posterior pillar since the palatopharyngeus muscle is involved in the sphincteric action of velopharyngeal closure. Undoubtedly, however, such cases are clinically rare. At any rate, the primary symptom associated with faucial abnormalities is proper oral-nasal resonance. Of course, it is also possible that in cases of hyperdistended tonsils, posterior tongue movement may be so restricted as to interfere with normal linguavelar articulations. Such potential difficulty should be noted by the examiner for later reference when considering the client's articulation defect. Faucial problems, especially with the tonsillar tissue, are typically of short duration. The lymphoid tissue decreases in size after puberty. Problems with the fauces should be referred to the client's physician, especially if they are of sufficient magnitude to interfere with speech.

Neck and Larynx

A thorough oral peripheral examination should include a general assessment of the functional integrity of the larynx and neck musculature. Disturbances in muscular tonicity in the region of the larynx and neck area may be observable in severe cases or may be detected by palpating the area. The speech pathologist should be alert to any conditions of muscular hypo- or hypertonicity. In cases of the latter, excessive muscular tension may be observable or palpable either at rest or during phonation. The larynx may be unusually elevated or malpositioned. The quality of phonation may be harsh or have a strangled sound. In severe cases, the hypertonicity may be sufficiently severe to make normal phonation difficult or to interrupt phonation completely. In addition to quality disturbances, the pitch level may be inappropriately high or low and the client may manifest upward or downward pitch breaks.

In clients with hypotonicity of the neck musculature, the maintenance of normal head posture may be difficult. The examiner may check the integrity of the neck muscles by placing his hand against the side of the client's head and asking him to resist the pressure. The procedure should be repeated on the opposite side, as well as in the front and back. The laryngeal musculature may be individually affected or may reflect a generalized pattern of head and neck paresis. In severe cases of laryngeal paralysis, the client may not be able to phonate at all. More commonly, the voice is weak and breathy as the result of incomplete vocal fold adduction and weakness. Of course, this condition must be differentiated from other laryngeal pathologies that may result in similar symptoms. The interested reader is referred to Boone (1977) for an indepth coverage of the topic.

The examiner will want to check the client's ability to sustain phonation and to start and stop phonation volitionally. A child should normally be able to sustain phonation for approximately ten seconds; an adult for approximately fifteen seconds. Repeated production of the vowel /a/ should be accomplished without effort.

Diadochokinesis

"Speech is a highly integrated physiologic act characterized by a series of complex motions executed in kinetic chains" (Fletcher, 1972). I have previously discussed the fact that normal speech production requires a structurally intact mechanism capable of fine motor coordinations. Deficits in neuromotor coordination may well lie at the heart of many articulation defects. Thus, the oral peripheral examination should routinely include an assessment of the client's ability to rapidly move the articulators in a manner requisite for speech articulation.

Diadochokinesis has traditionally been assessed by having the client produce nonsense syllables as rapidly as possible and by then computing the number of syllables produced over a given time period. This procedure requires that the examiner pay attention to both a stopwatch and the number of syllables produced. However, in 1972, Fletcher developed a "time-by-count" method that has simplified the process.

Rather than counting the number of syllable repetitions produced over, say, a five second time period, Fletcher suggests the use of time as the variable under measure. The client is asked to repeat a given nonsense syllable as rapidly as possible. The number of syllables is fixed (twenty repetitions of monosyllables; fifteen bisyllables; ten trisyllable productions). The examiner starts the stopwatch with the first syllable and stops it after the completion of the preestablished number of productions. The examiner then notes the total time required for the specific number of productions. The time required can then be compared to a table of norms, established for children from six to thirteen years of age. Table VI is taken from Fletcher's article and reveals the normative data he obtained from 384 children. Fletcher's article provides us with both means and standard deviations and makes it possible to calculate how far below the average a child might be in terms of diadochokinetic syllable rate.

Although Fletcher's data provide us with useful information, additional research is required to specify the exact significance of a given deviation in diadochokinesis. For example, how far below the mean must a child be before it becomes a potentially

TABLE VI
DIADOCHOKINETIC NORMS: MEAN TIME IN SECONDS REQUIRED FOR
CHILDREN TO PRODUCE 20 REPETITIONS OF THE MONOSYLLABLES, 15 OF
THE BISYLLABLES AND 10 OF THE TRISYLLABLE

Age	pʌ	tʌ	kʌ	fʌ	lʌ	pʌtə	pʌkə	tʌkə	pʌtəkə
6	4.8	4.9	5.5	5.5	5.2	7.3	7.9	7.8	10.3
7	4.8	4.9	5.3	5.4	5.3	7.6	8.0	8.0	10.0
8	4.2	4.4	4.8	4.9	4.6	6.2	7.1	7.2	8.3
9	4.0	4.1	4.6	4.6	4.5	5.9	6.6	6.6	7.7
10	3.7	3.8	4.3	4.2	4.2	5.5	6.4	6.4	7.1
11	3.6	3.6	4.0	4.0	3.8	4.8	5.8	5.8	6.5
12	3.4	3.5	3.9	3.7	3.7	4.7	5.7	5.5	6.4
13	3.3	3.3	3.7	3.6	3.5	4.2	5.1	5.1	5.7

SOURCE: Samuel G. Fletcher, Time-by-count measurement of diadochokinetic syllable rate, *Journal of Speech and Hearing Research*, 15:763-770, 1972.

significant finding? The author is presently engaged in a study designed to determine the relationships between specific diadochokinetic syllable rates and varying degrees of articulation defectiveness. Hopefully, the information will soon be available and will add to the diagnostic and prognostic significance of diadochokinetic assessment. At present, diadochokinetic assessment, using Fletcher's method, may provide the clinician with useful information concerning a client's relative articulatory mobility.

Articulatory sluggishness or incoordination may account for a fair percentage of the speech pathologist's articulatory defective caseload. As discussed in Chapter 2, there is ample evidence to support a fairly strong relationship between articulation defectiveness and poor fine motor skill development. There can be no question that clients with obvious neurological impairment may have articulation defects secondary to articulatory paralysis or incoordination (dysarthria in brain damaged adults or cerebral palsied children). However, many children with supposedly "functional" disorders also evidence poor oral motor control and reduced diadochokinesis (McNutt, 1977; Yoss and Darley, 1974).

The author suspects that many (perhaps 50%) of the children with articulation disorders may have underlying problems with oral sensory perception and oral motor control. This is probably especially true in clients with multiple misarticulations who evidence a high incidence of distortion errors. For the purpose of appropriate therapy planning, it is important to identify these children. Diadochokinetic assessment should be an integral part of the oral peripheral examination.

TRADITIONAL TESTS OF ARTICULATION

Traditional articulation tests are designed to sample a client's ability to produce the phonemes of our language. Each phoneme is usually tested in the initial, medial, and final position of single words. Single word responses are typically elicited by having the client name pictures presented by the examiner. However, tests and testing procedures may vary significantly. For example, a few commercially available tests sample a client's ability to produce the phonemes in the initial and final position of words only. Others employ objects, rather than pictures, to elicit responses, and some speech pathologists employ an imitative, rather than spontaneous (picture or object elicited), response mode.

The specific test or testing procedure employed is typically based on the examiner's purpose in testing. For instance, the choice of an imitative or spontaneous response mode should be made on the basis of whether the purpose is to simply identify error phonemes (screening) or to both identify the error phonemes and analyze the error pattern (diagnostic).

While there has been substantial controversy concerning the merits of these two procedures, the general consensus seems to be that the spontaneous method provides a sample that is more representative of the types of errors made in spontaneous, connected speech (Darley and Spriestersbach, 1978). However, having the client simply imitate the examiner's productions of the words is more economical of time and when the purpose is to identify phonemes in error in a large number of children, the imitative method may be preferred. In a recent study by Paynter and Bumpas (1978), the number of errors that three-year-old children made under imitative and spontaneous testing methods did not differ. However, the types of errors were found to be different and the authors conclude that "if the examiner is interested in the type of error or in doing a transcription of errors to determine error patterns, it would be better to use the spontaneous method of stimulus presentation."

Tests also vary in terms of the words and stimulus pictures used. Some consideration should, therefore, be given to the relative difficulty of the stimulus items in terms of the client's age, vocabulary, and ability to identify the pictures. Valuable clinical time may be wasted if the client is not able to spontaneously identify many of the stimulus pictures. Some tests will specify the age ranges that they were designed to sample; others will not.

In a recent study by Mullen and Whitehead (1978), the ability of children to recognize and identify the stimulus pictures on two different tests of articulation, the Goldman-Fristoe Test and the Arizona Articulation Proficiency Scale, was examined. They report that "the Arizona Test elicits significantly more correct initial stimulus picture identifications than does the Goldman-Fristoe Test." This should not be interpreted as suggesting that the Arizona is inherently a "better" test than the Goldman-Fristoe. It does, however, point out that the examiner should be alert to possible problems in stimulus picture identification with different tests, especially when testing younger clients.

In addition to the above, commercially available tests will vary in the number of phonemes that they sample and the number and type of phonetic contexts in which they are housed. While most tests include all of the consonant phonemes, some (screening tests) sample only the consonants most frequently misarticulated by children. Many tests include the cardinal vowels and diphthongs; some do not. While most test the consonants both as singletons and as elements in blends (clusters), the number of blends and types of consonant clusters vary from one test to another. Other tests are designed to sample only the phonemes that require high levels of intraoral breath pressure for correct production. These "pressure" tests are selected for clients with cleft palate or suspected velopharyngeal inadequacy.

Another difference among tests concerns the arrangement or ordering of the phonemes to be sampled. Some arrange the consonants in terms of phonemic groups, others according to place of articulation, and some according to the primary articulators concerned with their production. Such arrangements are designed to facilitate error analysis and to make identification of feature errors easier. Other tests list the target phonemes in the order in which they are supposedly mastered by the child. This provides a clearer picture of the child's developmental articulatory proficiency. However, in this respect, most articulation tests provide normative data with instructions on how to calculate an approximate "articulation age" based on the number of errors manifest or provide "cutoff" scores that suggest how many errors are acceptable (within normal limits) for a child of a given age. The author, however, urges caution in using such data. For the most part they concern number of errors alone and do not take into consideration the type or nature of the errors. For instance, while a certain number of sound substitutions characterized by single distinctive feature errors may be normal at certain ages, errors that are off-target by many features may not be considered developmentally normal.

Thus, the speech pathologist has many choices and considerations to make in selecting a test of articulation for clinical use. Considerations such as the number of phonemes sampled, the contexts in which they occur, the appropriateness of the stimulus words relative to the age and maturity of the clients being tested, whether or not to use a spontaneous response mode, the availability and type of normative data provided, and the arrangement of the test phonemes on the recording sheet should be given attention. There are numerous excellent tests commercially available. Darley and Spriestersbach (1978) and Nicolosi, Harryman, and Kresheck (1978) provide summary descriptions of most of the more widely used tests.

Figure 1 shows the Photo Articulation Test Recording Sheet. It was selected for illustrative purposes as a representative example of traditional tests of articulation. Inspection reveals that the target phonemes, listed in the left hand column, are categorized in terms of (I) lingual consonants, (II) labial consonants, and (III) vowels or diphthongs. Each consonant phoneme is tested in the initial, medial, and final position of the words shown in the second column. Spontaneous productions are elicited using color photographs of the objects. The /s/, /l/, and /r/ phonemes are tested as singletons and in blends. Fourteen vowels and four diphtongs are tested using some of the same words

					Year	Month	Day
Name_____		Date			____	____	____
School_____		Birth			____	____	____
Grade_____		Age			____	____	____

Key: Omission (–); substitution (write phonetic symbol of sound substituted); severity of distortion (D1), (D2), (D3); ability to imitate (circle symbol or error).

Sound	Photograph	1	2	3	Vowels, Diph.		Comments
	I				**III**		
s	saw, pencil, house				aʊ	house	
s bl	spoon, skates, stars						
z	zipper, scissors, keys						
ʃ	shoe, station, fish				u	shoe	
tʃ	chair, matches, sandwich						
dʒ	jars, angels, orange						
t	table, potatoes, hat				æ	hat	
d	dog, ladder, bed				ɔ	dog	
n	nails, bananas, can				ə	bananas	
l	lamp, balloons, bell				ɛ	bell	
l bl	blocks, clock, flag				ɑ	blocks	
θ	thumb, toothbrush, teeth				i	teeth	
r	radio, carrots, car						
r bl	brush, crayons, train				e	train	
k	cat, crackers, cake				ɚ-ə	crackers	
g	gun, wagon, egg				ʌ	gun	
	II						
f	fork, elephant, knife						
v	vacuum, TV, stove				ju	vacuum	
p	pipe, apples, cup				aɪ	pipe	
b	book, baby, bathtub				ʊ	book	
m	monkey, hammer, comb				o	comb	**SCORE**
w-hw	witch, flowers, whistle				ɪ	witch	
	I						*Sounds*
ð	this, that, feathers, bathe						I Tongue_____
h-ŋ	hanger, hanger, swing						II Lip _____
j	yes, thank you						III Vowels_____
ʒ	measure, beige				ɔɪ	boy	Total _____
	(story)				ɝ-ɜ	bird	

Figure 1. PAT RECORDING SHEET. From K. Pendergast, S. Dickey, J. Selmar, and A. Soder, *Photo Articulation Test*, 1969. Courtesy of The Interstate Printers and Publisher, Inc., Danville, Illinois.

designed to test the consonants. For example, the client's production of the stimulus word "house" allows the examiner to test both the final /s/ and the diphthong /au/. The client's responses are recorded in the spaces provided. The numbers 1, 2, and 3 designate the phoneme's position in the words; initial, medial, and final, respectively.

Substitution errors are transcribed using the proper phonetic symbol of the sound produced. Omission errors are symbolized by drawing a horizontal slash through the appropriate space and distortion errors are noted as D1, D2, or D3, relative to the degree of severity of the error (degree to which the phonetic deviation fails to approximate the target phoneme). However, it should be remembered that distortion errors are, in reality, nonphonemic substitutions and it is important that the specific nature of the errors be identified as closely as possible.

For this reason, it is suggested that the examiner, regardless of the test being used, describe the distortion errors in terms of physiological phonetics. In planning therapy, it is important to know the exact nature of the client's errors and what he is doing incorrectly in his attempt to produce the target sounds. Thus, the examiner may designate a distortion error using the suggested symbol "D" and then describe the nature of the misarticulation in either the Comments Section or in an addendum to the recording sheet. An alternate way would be to establish an arbitrary symbol that describes a particular distortion error and to note it in a legend somewhere on the sheet. The symbol could then be used to designate the nonphonemic substitution error whenever it occurred. For example, we might use the symbol /ʃ/ to designate a lateral lisp. Once we noted the symbol and its description in the legend we could use it in the spaces provided to represent the error. Multiple different distortion errors might be more efficiently recorded in this manner.

Regardless of the specific test selected, traditional tests provide us with useful clinical information. From the test results we can determine, (1) how many sounds are incorrectly produced; (2) which sounds are defective; (3) the prevalent error pattern with reference to type, i.e. omissions, substitutions, distortions; and (4) the prevalent error pattern with reference to position, i.e. initial, medial, or final location within words. Such information is undoubtedly useful in providing the clinician with pre-liminary indications of the severity and magnitude of the disorder, as well as the basic pattern of the client's faulty articulation.

As a general rule of thumb, the greater the number of errors the more severe the problem. Also, as discussed in Chapter 4, omission errors are considered to be more severe than substitution errors and a prevalent substitution error pattern is typically, although not always, indicative of a more severe problem than one involving primarily distortion errors. An obvious exception can be found in clients with dysarthria. In such clients a prevalent distortion error pattern is common due to neuromotor paralysis or incoordination. Such errors are frequently more severe than phonemic substitutions since they are more resistant to correction.

A consideration of the specific phonemes in error also allows an estimate of the magnitude of the problem. Misarticulation of the phonemes that are normally mastered earlier in the developmental sequence would constitute a more serious problem than misarticulations involving only the developmentally more advanced phonemes. Misarticulation of the phonemes that occur more often in connected speech would represent a more severe defect than misarticulations involving phonemes with a low frequency of occurrence. Finally, the prevalent place of misarticulation (initial, medial, or final position) in the word might contribute severity information. Although not as certain as some of the above information, errors in the initial position of single words tend to draw a little more attention than errors involving the final position. Omission errors are more common in the final position. Thus, errors in the initial position may be considered somewhat more severe, all other things being equal.

In addition to the information above, traditional articulation tests provide an excellent framework for stimulability testing. After completing the articulation test the client should be checked for stimulability on each of the error sounds. As discussed in Chapter 4, stimulability information is important in considering severity, prognosis, and planning therapy and is easily obtainable. It is traditionally tested by having the client attempt to imitate an identified error sound after the clinician has instructed the client to watch and listen closely to the sound modeled in isolation. Of course it may also be tested by modeling the sound in words in the position(s) in which it was found to be in error on the articulation test.

For useful therapy information it is probably best to also check stimulability when a visual or auditory model only is provided. Compared with the traditional "Watch me and listen carefully" approach, the information may provide insight concerning the most effective modality for stimulus presentation in therapy (visual alone, auditory alone, or auditory-visual approach). For the same reason, if the client is not found to be stimulable using any of the above procedures, the clinician should couple the auditory-visual model with some phonetic instruction concerning the placement of the articulators. Error sounds on which the client is stimulable may be circled on the articulation score sheet with a notation made concerning the method of stimulation. Error sounds that are highly stimulable are generally more amenable to correction than those with low stimulability.

In recent years the validity of traditional articulation testing as a method of sampling a client's speech has been called into question. The issue concerns the degree to which speech sound production elicited via picture naming is representative of speech sound production in connected spontaneous speech. As the reader will recall from the discussion on coarticulation in Chapter 1, in connected speech the speaker does not produce individual autonomous phonemes, or even phones for that matter. Rather, the target values for each phone (phoneme at a mentalistic level) are modified to varying degrees as a result of the interaction or coarticulation with neighboring phones. This allophonic variation is primarily the result of phonetic context. Thus, many have objected to the use of picture-elicited, single word tests on the following grounds: (1) three single word responses do not provide a sufficiently representative sample considering the number of phonetic contexts and allophonic variation in connected speech and (2) just as phonemes are not produced as separate entities, neither are single words in connected speech.

A number of investigators have studied the question by comparing the results of traditional testing with those obtained by eliciting connected speech samples (Faircloth and Faircloth,

1970; Hutchinson, 1972; Dubois and Bernthal, 1978). The studies by Faircloth and Faircloth and by Dubois and Bernthal reveal that clients make more errors in connected speech than they do in producing isolated single words. Thus, one problem with traditional testing methods is that the speech pathologist may fail to identify certain sound errors that are present in the client's spontaneous connected speech. Another possibility is that the exact nature of the errors may differ across phonetic contexts in connected speech. Such variation in error type may not be apparent from traditional test results.

It would appear that most of the authors of traditional articulation tests have acknowledged the potential limitations since the majority attempt to compensate for them. For example, some tests list additional test words in their appendices, designed to assist the examiner in sampling the consistency of a particular error and, at the same time, providing additional phonetic contexts in which to sample the sound. Others encourage examiners to obtain a connected speech sample following test administration and to compare the identified errors with those in the connected sample. Some tests have written material to be read or pictures to be described by the client, expressly for the purpose of obtaining a connected speech sample.

While these reflect gallant attempts to improve the validity of the test results, they typically fall short in terms of systematically obtaining a completely representative sample of the client's connected speech. However, as described above, traditional single word tests are of clinical value and should not be discarded. It is apparent though that additional testing is needed in order to determine the influence of different phonetic contexts on an identified error and to assess error consistency. It was for this purpose that McDonald (1964) developed the Deep Test of Articulation.

DEEP TESTS OF ARTICULATION

In 1964, McDonald published a text on articulation testing and treatment that emphasizes the physiological, phonetic nature of speech. He suggests that at the physical level of speech the primary unit of production is the syllable, not the word. Using the syllable as a frame of reference, McDonald describes the roles or functions of consonants and vowels. He suggests that vowels function to shape the vocal tract, i.e. account for its primary configuration, and that consonants function to either *release* or *arrest* the syllable unit. Thus, in the word (syllable) "cat," the vowel /æ/ gives the vocal tract its characteristic shape, the consonant /k/ functions to release the syllable and the consonant /t/ functions as the syllable arrestor.

The focus on the syllable as the primary unit of speech production and the description of consonants in terms of releasing or arresting the syllable pulse are more consistent with physiological reality than the traditional view of consonants occurring in the initial, medial, or final position of single words. Viewing the syllable as the fundamental unit of speech production makes the use of the terms *initial, medial,* and *final* inappropriate. Although it might be possible to think of releasing consonant as occurring in the initial position of a syllable and an arresting consonant as occurring in the final position, the "medial" position would be totally irrelevant. For example, in the word "pencil," the word used in the Photo Articulation Test to sample the /s/ in the "medial" position, we actually produce two syllables (pen and cil). In this case, the /s/ is functioning to release the second syllable or, in terms of position, occurs in the initial position of the syllable.

Similarly, in the word "bathtub," a word commonly used to test the "medial" /θ/, the /θ/ actually serves to arrest the first syllable "bath" or, we might say that it occurs in the final position of the syllable. From this we might logically assume that sound errors occurring on phonemes in the purported medial position of single words (traditional test) should be the same as those occurring on sounds in either the initial or final positions depending upon whether the test consonant actually serves to release (initial) or arrest (final) the syllable. This assumption is consistent with the author's clinical experience, although there is occasionally some variability attributable to differences in phonetic context.

As discussed in Chapter 1, the production of a sound is modified according to phonetic context. Coarticulation effects may greatly influence the ease with which we are able to achieve or approximate certain articulatory targets that may be distinctive for a given phoneme. Therefore, a client may articulate a sound correctly in one context but miss the salient target(s) in another. This may account for a large part of what we label *inconsistency* in reference to a client's error sounds. McDonald suggests that it is important to systematically examine the influence of phonetic context on an identified error sound in order to (1) determine the degree of consistency of the error and (2) identify those phonetic contexts in which the client is able to correctly articulate the sound. Those contexts in which the sound is produced correctly are referred to as *facilitory contexts* and their identification may provide useful information for therapy planning.

From the above, it should be clear to the reader that, at the level of production there are as many variations of a sound (allophones) as there are phonetic contexts. This reasoning led McDonald to suggest that an adequate test of a speaker's ability to produce a given phone would require that the phone be sampled in a representative number of phonetic contexts. Traditional tests of articulation are inadequate in this respect since they sample a given phone in only two or three contexts.

McDonald's *Deep Test of Articulation* (1964) is designed to assess identified error sounds in a representative sample of phonetic contexts. Consonant error sounds are tested intersyllabically as they function first to release the second syllable and then to arrest the first syllable. Thirty contexts are provided for assessing the identified error phone. While the test booklets provide ample instruction on test administration, a brief description might help the reader better understand the constructs.

The Deep Test has two forms: a sentence form for older children and adults and a picture form for younger children who are not proficient readers. The picture form consists of a series of plates that picture easily recognized monosyllable words. Two plates (pictures) are presented to the child simultaneously (side by side) and he is asked to "make one big funny word" out of the two.

For example, in practice trials, the child may be shown a picture of a bat and a picture of a man. By making one word out of the two, it would be possible to assess the abutting consonants /t/ and /m/ and to determine their reciprocal influence on each other. In this practice trial example, the /t/ could be tested as it functioned to arrest the syllable "bat" and in the abutting context of /m/ or the /m/ could be tested as a syllable releasor as it abutted with /t/.

Once the child is proficient at the task of combining the monosyllable words in a "connected speech manner" (several practice plates are provided), the examiner may begin testing a particular error sound. The phone would first be tested as it functioned to release a monosyllable word and then as it served to arrest a monosyllable. For example, if the /s/ were the test phone, the plate depicting a picture of the sun would be used to test the sound as a syllable releasor. The child would then be shown all of the pictures on the left hand side of the booklet and asked to combine them with the word "sun." The accuracy or type of error(s) made on the /s/ would be appropriately noted on the record sheet.

To test the /s/ as a syllable arrestor, a plate depicting a picture of a house is used and the word is abutted with all the plates on the right hand side of the booklet. Errors or correct productions of the /s/ are again noted in the proper column on the record sheet. In this manner, error sounds are tested as syllable arrestors and releasors in a wide variety of phonetic contexts.

Figure 2 shows a copy of the Deep Test Record Sheet. As noted in the instructions at the top of the sheet, the test phoneme is placed in the bracket at the top of a column. Four brackets and columns are available for either testing four different phonemes or for retesting a single phoneme on different dates. The blanks on the left hand side of the column are for recording the client's productions of the test sound when it functions to release a monosyllable while those on the right hand side provide for scoring the sound when it serves to arrest a monosyllable.

Analysis of the Deep Test results may provide valuable clinical information. An overall index of error consistency may be obtained by dividing the total number of errors by the total number of productions elicited (not all phonetic contexts can be tested) and by multiplying the quotient by 100. As discussed in Chapter 4, error consistency provides us with information concerning severity and prognosis. Error sounds that are highly consistent are more firmly established in the client's repertoire and are

Instructions: Within the brackets write the phonetic symbol for the sound deep tested, e.g.,[s]. Use the symbols you prefer to indicate whether the sound was articulated correctly or the nature of the incorrect articulation (substitution, omission, or distortion) for each of the indicated phonetic contexts. Not all phonetic contexts can be tested. To determine the percent of correct articulations, divide the number of *correct* responses by the number of phonemes tested and multiply the quotient by 100.

INDIVIDUAL RECORD SHEET for a DEEP TEST OF ARTICULATION

Name — Age — Grade — Date

Address or School — Test used: — Picture — Sentence

Tester

[ ]	[ ]	[ ]	[ ]
*			
p — 1 — p	p — 1 — p	p — 1 — p	p — 1 — p
b — 2 — b	b — 2 — b	b — 2 — b	b — 2 — b
t — 3 — t	t — 3 — t	t — 3 — t	t — 3 — t
d — 4 — d	d — 4 — d	d — 4 — d	d — 4 — d
k — 5 — k	k — 5 — k	k — 5 — k	k — 5 — k
g — 6 — g	g — 6 — g	g — 6 — g	g — 6 — g
m — 7 — m	m — 7 — m	m — 7 — m	m — 7 — m
n — 8 — n	n — 8 — n	n — 8 — n	n — 8 — n
f — 9 — f	f — 9 — f	f — 9 — f	f — 9 — f
v — 10 — v	v — 10 — v	v — 10 — v	v — 10 — v
θ — 11 — θ	θ — 11 — θ	θ — 11 — θ	θ — 11 — θ
ð — 12 — ð	ð — 12 — ð	ð — 12 — ð	ð — 12 — ð
s — 13 — s	s — 13 — s	s — 13 — s	s — 13 — s
z — 14 — z	z — 14 — z	z — 14 — z	z — 14 — z
ʃ — 15 — ʃ	ʃ — 15 — ʃ	ʃ — 15 — ʃ	ʃ — 15 — ʃ
tʃ — 16 — tʃ	tʃ — 16 — tʃ	tʃ — 16 — tʃ	tʃ — 16 — tʃ
dʒ — 17 — dʒ	dʒ — 17 — dʒ	dʒ — 17 — dʒ	dʒ — 17 — dʒ
l — 18 — l	l — 18 — l	l — 18 — l	l — 18 — l
r — 19 — r	r — 19 — r	r — 19 — r	r — 19 — r
j — 20 — j	j — 20 — j	j — 20 — j	j — 20 — j
w — 21 — w	w — 21 — w	w — 21 — w	w — 21 — w
h — 22 — h	h — 22 — h	h — 22 — h	h — 22 — h
ŋ — 23 — ŋ	ŋ — 23 — ŋ	ŋ — 23 — ŋ	ŋ — 23 — ŋ
i — 24 — i	i — 24 — i	i — 24 — i	i — 24 — i
ɪ — 25 — ɪ	ɪ — 25 — ɪ	ɪ — 25 — ɪ	ɪ — 25 — ɪ
ɛ — 26 — ɛ	ɛ — 26 — ɛ	ɛ — 26 — ɛ	ɛ — 26 — ɛ
æ — 27 — æ	æ — 27 — æ	æ — 27 — æ	æ — 27 — æ
ʌ — 28 — ʌ	ʌ — 28 — ʌ	ʌ — 28 — ʌ	ʌ — 28 — ʌ
u — 29 — u	u — 29 — u	u — 29 — u	u — 29 — u
ɔ — 30 — ɔ	ɔ — 30 — ɔ	ɔ — 30 — ɔ	ɔ — 30 — ɔ
%Correct	%Correct	%Correct	%Correct
Date Tested	Date Tested	Date Tested	Date Tested

*The numbers correspond to the sentence number or picture number in The Deep Test of Articulation

Figure 2. DEEP TEST RECORD SHEET. From Eugene T. McDonald, *Deep Test of Articulation,* 1964. Courtesy of Stanwix House, Inc., Pittsburgh, Pennsylvania.

generally more resistant to correction. On the other hand, highly inconsistent errors are typically not as firmly entrenched and are more easily corrected. In cases where a sound is defective in only a few environments, say, less than 10 or 20 percent of the time, the error stands a good chance of being corrected spontaneously and therapy for correction of the phoneme may not be warranted. Of course, research is needed to verify this clinical observation and, undoubtedly, other variables, such as the client's age and stimulability must also be taken into consideration. For example, it is probably unreasonable to assume that a client will spontaneously outgrow a highly inconsistent error if he is well past the expected age of developmental mastery and if he is not stimulable on the sound in the noted error contexts.

In addition to an overall index of error consistency, the Deep Test results may be analyzed to determine whether the errors occur primarily when the consonant functions to release or arrest the syllable. It is not at all uncommon to find that errors are restricted primarily to one category or the other and, as will be discussed in Chapter 4, this provides valuable information for planning therapy. As already mentioned, test results should also be analyzed in order to identify possible facilitory contexts. It is possible to use such information as the springboard for therapy.

The Deep Test provides an excellent tool for the phonetic assessment of identified error sounds. However, the reader must be wondering how to identify the error phonemes in the first place. Many practicing speech pathologists use a traditional, three position, single word articulation test for the purpose. Others have chosen to use the *Screening Deep Test of Articulation.* Developed by McDonald in 1968, the Screening Test assesses nine of the most frequently misarticulated phonemes by children. The phonemes tested are the /s/, /l/, /r/, /tʃ/, /θ/, /ʃ/, /k/, /f/ and /t/. Each phoneme is tested in ten different phonetic contexts. The format is roughly the same as that of the Deep Test, however, two to four phonemes may be tested in one production of the combined monosyllables.

Figure 3 shows a copy of the Screening Test Record Sheet and may help clarify the test for the reader. The Test consists of thirty-one plates. Each plate depicts two monosyllable words that the client is instructed to produce as one word. The first test

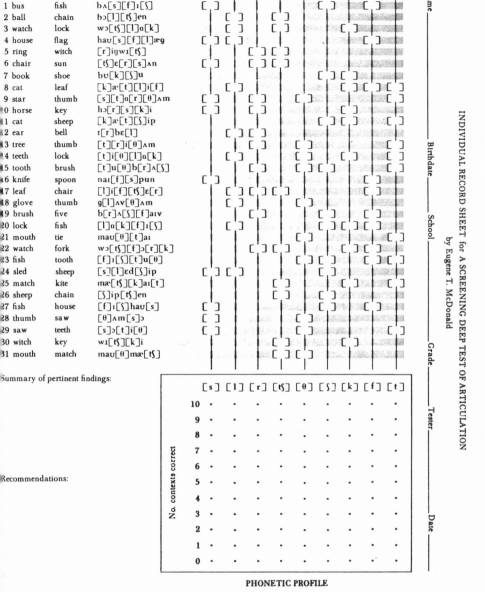

Figure 3. SCREENING DEEP TEST RECORD SHEET. From Eugene T. McDonald, *Screening Deep Test of Articulation,* 1968. Courtesy of Stanwix House, Inc., Pittsburgh, Pennsylvania.

plate contains the pictures of a bus and a fish. This item allows the examiner to test the phonemes /s/, /f/ and /ʃ/. After all thirty-one plates are administered, the clinician notes the number of instances (out of ten) in which the sound was produced correctly and circles the number in the Phonetic Profile box at the bottom of the Record Sheet. Thus, the Screening Test not only identifies specific error phonemes but also provides a rough estimate of consistency.

McDonald's Screening Deep Test is an excellent tool for screening large numbers of school-aged children. It can be administered in a short period of time and samples the most frequently misarticulated phonemes in a manner that more nearly approximates spontaneous connected speech. In addition, McDonald (1974, 1976) has established normative data for the Screening Test. The norms refer to the number of contexts in which sounds are correctly articulated by children in kindergarten through the beginning of the third grade. The data include cutoff scores relative to the need for administering the Deep Test at the various grade levels. Deep Test results then allow the speech pathologist to make a decision concerning the need for therapy. Such information should prove to be of great value to the public school clinician in making decisions concerning caseload selection, prognosis, and therapy.

By deep testing an error sound we are able to obtain information concerning the consistency with which a client misarticulates a phoneme. In addition to providing an index of severity and prognosis and rendering valuable therapy information, consistency data, as noted in Chapter 4, may provide one means of differentiating between phonetic and phonemic disorders. As the reader will recall, phonetically based disorders involve the actual articulomotor production of speech, that is, reflect a client's difficulty in directing the articulators toward and/or achieving the salient phonetic targets that are distinctively characteristic of a given phoneme. Phonemically based disorders, on the other hand, reflect a client's inability to differentiate between phonemes at a conceptual level, either due to his failure to acquire a given distinctive feature or a rule governing the correct selection and combination of one or more distinctive features that comprise a phoneme.

Phonetically based disorders are, in general, due to some form of structural or neuromotor deficiency. As such, we would not routinely expect to find much variability in the articulation errors across phonetic contexts. While a few phonetic contexts may prove to be facilitory with reference to the ease with which a specific target may be hit, we would generally expect a high error consistency. Therefore, a low or moderate percentage of error consistency more likely reflects a phonemically based disorder. The reasoning is that if a client possesses sufficient structural and neuromotor capability to produce the movements needed for correct articulation of a sound in a number of contexts, his errors in other contexts more likely reflect a misapplication of a feature combinatorial rule. In discussing the nature of a client's articulation disorder, Perkins (1977) states the following:

> Is the difficulty one of differentiating phonemic targets or one of being able to direct ballistic movements to the targets? If all necessary movements can be produced in some phonetic contexts but are not used in others, differentiation of the sounds would be expected. If some necessary movements are not achieved in any phonetic context, neuromuscular control would be suspected (p. 347).

DISTINCTIVE FEATURE ANALYSIS

If the reader were to follow the developmental chronology of this chapter in assessing a client, he would take a case history, complete an oral peripheral examination, administer a traditional test of articulation, assess error stimulability, administer the Deep Test of Articulation, and determine error consistency. From the traditional articulation test the clinician would be able to determine how many sounds were in error, identify the particular error phonemes, determine the prevalent error type (omissions, substitutions, distortions) and the location of the errors in words (initial, medial, or final position). From the Deep Test he would be able to identify facilitating phonetic contexts and determine whether errors occur primarily as syllable arrestors or releasors. Although the foregoing information may provide the clinician with clinical insight concerning the severity of the disorder, prognosis, the general nature of the problem, and tentative therapy planning, most speech pathologists go further in their assessment.

Once error sounds have been identified, the clinician should attempt to discern the nature of the errors and search for consistencies or the *defective feature pattern* that may underlie the manifest errors. Multiple articulation errors do not occur randomly. The client's error sounds, like his correct sounds, are rule governed. Several errors may share a common ingredient that accounts for their defectiveness. For example, the /t/, /d/, /l/, and /n/ phonemes may be in error because the child has not acquired the linguaalveolar place feature. Similarly, a single voice or manner feature may be the culprit underlying many sound errors. Thus, an analysis of the sound errors in terms of defective features may allow for delineation of the common factor(s) accounting for the errors. As discussed in Chapter 1, the identification of feature errors may aid the clinician in understanding the nature of the disorder and, as McReynolds and Huston (1971) suggest, may allow the clinician to develop a more efficient therapy plan. By identifying the subphonemic element (distinctive feature) that lies at the heart of many sound errors, clinicians may focus therapy on the defective element rather than working on each error sound separately. More will be said about this in the next chapter.

As reviewed in Chapter 1, there are numerous distinctive feature systems that the clinician may use in analyzing a client's defective articulation. At present there is no single universally endorsed system for use by the speech pathologist. There are, however, differences among systems. For example, systems such as those developed by Chomsky and Halle (1968) and Jakobson, Faut, and Halle (1951) (see Chapter 1 for review) are designed to be universally applicable across languages while others are specific to the English language. Systems vary in the number of features included and in their derivation, i.e. some have acoustic reference while others use articulatory or perceptual classifications. Some systems are completely binary (a given feature is either present or absent) while others are multivalued or have a combination of binary and multivalued features. Representative of the latter type are the place, manner, and voicing systems that most clinicians have been familiarized with during their introductory phonetics training.

McReynolds (1977) suggests that phonemic errors may be

analyzed using a number of systems but that "the particular system used or selected depends upon the clinician's need for specificity." For example, she suggests that a "place and manner" system might be more appropriate for analyzing a child's misarticulations when the sound errors consist of many place feature errors. The rationale is that the place and manner systems typically contain more place designations and, therefore, can provide more delineating specific information.

As implied in Chapter 1, the place, manner, and voicing systems have traditionally been referred to as *phonetic* feature systems. Table II, in the first chapter, is labelled as a phonetic feature matrix. The term *phonetic* is used to suggest that the features have a direct articulatory reference and refer to the production of English sounds. The term has, undoubtedly, been carried over from the use of such classification systems in doing "phonetic analyses" prior to the advent of distinctive feature theory. However, the reader should understand that such systems are, in reality, phonemic. While the features in these systems may not be completely binary, they do refer to idealized targets or production values (place, manner, and voicing) that allow one phoneme to be differentiated from another. This is simply to say that such systems are comprised of phonemically distinctive features and, as such, are not inherently different from other linguistic systems discussed in Chapter 1.

Pending further research on new developments in the applications of distinctive feature theory, it is the author's present belief that place, manner, and voicing systems offer the clinician the best vehicle for identifying error patterns and planning remediation. Such systems typically allow greater specificity with regard to place errors and afford a clear articulatory reference to manner errors. While distinctive feature systems are not, by nature, typically applicable to the assessment of nonphonemic errors (distortions), the greater degree of place specificity and articulatory reference in the place, manner, and voicing systems make it possible to analyze many of these errors.

Place, manner, and voicing systems vary substantially in the number of features used. They may contain only a few features or may be more elaborate in number and phonetic detail. An example of the latter may be found in the feature system developed by Walsh (1974). Again, the selection of a given feature system depends upon the clinician's need for specificity.

The mechanics of doing a feature analysis are rather straightforward. Several examples may be found in the literature (McReynolds and Engmann, 1975; Singh, 1976; Turton, 1973). Basically, it involves comparing the features comprising the target phoneme with the features actually produced in the replacement phoneme. The features or feature designations that are not shared by the two phonemes are noted as feature errors. By specifying the feature errors across multiple phoneme errors it may be possible to discern a pattern.

To demonstrate the process, let us assume that we have administered a traditional articulation test to a child and have identified the following phoneme errors: t/s; d/z; t/ʃ; d/ʒ; p/f; and b/v. We may analyze these errors using the feature system outlined in Table II in the first chapter.

Table VII shows a feature analysis of these errors. Examination of Table VII may help the reader better understand the process. The place, manner, and voicing features or designations are listed in the left-hand column. The notations "E/T" at the top of the Table designate the error or replacement phoneme (E) and target phoneme (T), respectively. The child's substitution errors (/t/ for /s/, /d/ for /z/, etc.) are noted under the "E/T" headings. The specific place, manner, and voicing features comprising the replacement and target phonemes are noted in the columns with a plus (+) indicating that the feature is present and a minus (−) indicating the absence of a feature. While the system is not truly binary, the plus-minus markings were chosen as a convenient method to designate the "feature bundles" comprising the phonemes. By noting the feature differences between the target and error phonemes we may specify the exact nature of the substitution errors.

At the bottom of the Table we may note the number of feature errors per phoneme error. It should be noted that although there are fourteen features in the system, a maximum of only three feature errors is possible, i.e. place, manner, and voicing. This is because of the multivalued nature of the system. The total number of the place, manner, and voicing errors may be found

TABLE VII
SAMPLE FEATURE ANALYSIS

Features	E/T	E/T	E/T	E/T	E/T	E/T	Errors
	t/s	d/z	t/ʃ	d/ʒ	p/f	b/v	
Place							
labial	− −	− −	− −	− −	+ −	+ −	labial/labiodental
labiodental	− −	− −	− −	− −	− +	− +	
linguadental	− −	− −	− −	− −	− −	− −	
alveolar	+ +	+ +	+ −	+ −	− −	− −	alveolar/palatal
palatal	− −	− −	− +	− +	− −	− −	
velar	− −	− −	− −	− −	− −	− −	
glottal	− −	− −	− −	− −	− −	− −	
Manner							
nasal	− −	− −	− −	− −	− −	− −	
plosive	+ −	+ −	+ −	+ −	+ −	+ −	plosive/fricative
fricative	− +	− +	− +	− +	− +	− +	
affricate	− −	− −	− −	− −	− −	− −	
liquid	− −	− −	− −	− −	− −	− −	
glide	− −	− −	− −	− −	− −	− −	
Voicing	− −	+ +	− −	+ +	− −	+ +	

Errors								
Place	=			×	×	×	×	4
Manner	=	×	×	×	×	×	×	6
Voicing	=							0
Total	=	1	1	2	2	2	2	10

in the lower right-hand corner of the Table. Combined, these data provide us with information concerning severity.

As discussed in Chapter 1, a larger number of feature errors in a given substitution suggests a more severe error. This is to say that a sound substitution error that is different from the target phoneme by only one feature, for example place of articulation, is less severe than a substitution that is off-target in terms of place, manner, and voicing. Similarly, a larger number of total feature errors generally suggests a more severe articulation defect.

In analyzing our hypothetical child's misarticulations we can see that all six phoneme errors are characterized by manner errors. Specifically, the child is substituting a plosive for a fricative in all six phonemes. Four of the phoneme substitutions involve place feature errors. Alveolars replace palatals in the t/ʃ and d/ʒ errors and labials replace labiodentals in the p/f and b/v substitutions. However, the place feature errors are probably an artifact of the manner substitutions. The child is substituting plosives for fricatives. There are no plosives with either palatal or labiodental place specifications. Thus, the child appears to have selected replacement plosives with the place feature closest to that of the target fricative. Based on the above it is possible to specify the *error rules* with which the child is apparently operating: (1) substitute plosive phonemes for the fricatives /s/, /z/, /ʃ/, /ʒ/, /f/, and /v/ and (2) when a replacement plosive with the same place feature is unavailable, select the plosive with the closest anterior place designation.

It should be mentioned that our hypothetical child has the concept of "frication" since the feature appears in his correct productions of the fricative phonemes /θ/, /ð/, /h/ and /hw/. Thus, the problem would appear to be one of rule generalization. While the fricative feature appears in his repertoire, the child has not learned to combine the feature with the feature bundles comprising the defective phonemes. For an indepth discussion of the analysis of children's deviant phonological rules, the reader is referred to Ingram's excellent 1976 publication on the subject.

As suggested in previous sections of this chapter, children are frequently inconsistent in the substitutions that they use for a given defective phoneme. The nature of such inconsistency may be revealed from deep testing. In cases where more than one replacement phoneme is used by the child, the clinician may undertake multiple feature analyses and then specify the child's error rules in terms of the surrounding phonetic or phonemic contexts. It may be that a specific feature will appear in certain phonetic or positional contexts but not in others. The reader is referred to a publication by Standel, Gardner, and Hannah (1977) for one example of how to analyze multiple substitutions involving a single phoneme.

Singh (1976) reports that Singh and Frank, in a 1972 study, did distinctive feature analyses of the defective articulation of ninety children. Based on their findings, they were able to discern some consistencies in children's deviant phonological rules. Those consistencies are summarized as follows:

1. The most recently acquired phonemes are replaced most often.
2. Phonemes used as substitutes are most often the ones learned earliest.
3. The stop feature is the most frequent replacement for other manner features:
   a. fricatives and nasals are replaced by stops
   b. stops are not replaced
   c. nasals and fricatives do not substitute for each other.
4. A place feature is substituted by the closest more frontal place in the same manner of articulation:
   a. alveolar replaces back
   b. interdental replaces alveolar
   c. labial replaces alveolar.
5. If the closest, more frontal feature has not yet emerged in the same manner series, then there is a change in both the place and manner series.
   For example, according to rule 4a, /ʃ/ is replaced by /s/. However, if /s/ has not appeared in the child's repertoire, /ʃ/ is replaced by /t/.
6. Voiceless more frequently substitutes the voiced feature than vice versa.
7. Substitutions are influenced by stability and similarity of phonemes (p. 217).

These conclusions are consistent with the author's clinical observations and certainly applicable to our hypothetical child's deviant rule system.

SPEECH SOUND DISCRIMINATION

The ability of a child to perceive the differences between speech sounds is obviously vital to phonemic development. If unable to distinguish the feature difference(s) between two phonemes, a child will perceive and produce them as one. An integral component in the child's phonological development is a progressive refinement in his ability to detect and discriminate among the phonemes of English in terms of their distinctive feature characteristics. As discussed in Chapter 2, Menyuk (1968) suggests that the phonemes acquired earliest in the child's development are those containing features that are the most readily discriminable. Phonemes typically mastered later in the developmental sequence contain more difficult to discriminate features. Tannahill and McReynolds (1972) suggest that phonemes containing many feature differences are easier to discriminate than phoneme pairs having only a single feature difference.

As suggested in Chapter 2, the majority of clients with articulation disorders have at least some degree of difficulty in auditorily discriminating between speech sounds. Those with more severe articulation defects tend to show more generalized deficits while those with only a few misarticulations appear to have more specific discrimination difficulty involving their error sounds only. Although there are undoubtedly exceptions to this general observation, it appears to be a reasonably valid "rule of thumb" and consistent with clinical experience.

The results obtained in discrimination testing are heavily influenced by the testing paradigm employed. Different test protocols may actually examine different levels of discrimination processing and may represent inherently different degrees of difficulty. Three different test protocols, which in the author's opinion reflect different levels of processing and difficulty, are described below. They are arranged in order from the least to the most difficult.

1. *The External-External Format* is probably the most commonly employed in discrimination testing. Wepman's Auditory Discrimination Test (1973) is of this type. The typical test procedure involves having the client, seated facing away from the examiner, listen to pairs of words read by the examiner and indicate whether the word pairs are the same (a single word repeated) or different (two different words). The words are typically CVCs and differ by a single phoneme; for example, hat-pat, pass-path, etc. Prior to testing the child should be tested to make certain that the concepts of same-different are within his repertoire. Alternate terms, such as alike or not alike, may be used.

The clinician may design his own test and then analyze the client's errors in terms of the specific phoneme-feature confusions. Tests may be administered in quiet or under various conditions of noise. The advantage of a clinician designed test is that minimal word pairs may be selected that examine the particular phoneme or feature contrasts contained in the client's production errors. The errors may be analyzed to determine whether a generalized or specific discrimination deficit exists. The primary advantage in using a standardized test such as

Wepman's is that normative data are provided that allow the clinician to compare the client's correct number of responses with those of other children his own age. Wepman's normative data allow a direct estimate of the magnitude of the problem. Interestingly, the upper age level in Wepman's norms is eight years, since "above the age of 8 almost no change is found in auditory discrimination ability."

This type of testing is referred to as external-external since both stimuli are presented by an external source — the examiner. The child's performance on such a test may provide useful information, however, many children will show normal ability on such a test and yet have a discrimination deficit.

2. *The External-Internal Format* is designed to assess the client's ability to compare his own productions with those of others. The client typically has more difficulty with this type of task, especially when the comparisons involve his error sounds. Specific test procedures vary. Some clinicians use an imitation procedure in which they produce a series of words, many containing the child's error sounds. After each production the child says the word and is then asked if his production was the same as the clinician's. Another procedure, preferred by the author, is to have the client name stimulus pictures. Following each response, the clinician produces the word and asks the client to make a judgment of same or different. In cases where the stimulus words contain an error phoneme, the clinician may vary his productions, sometimes producing it in error like the client and sometimes producing it correctly. Regardless of the exact procedure employed, the results of such testing may reveal the degree to which a client is able to recognize that his productions are different from the standard. Such information is highly valuable in considering the initial design of therapy.

3. *The Internal-Internal Format* refers to the assessment of client's self-monitoring ability. The client is asked to name stimulus pictures or to describe a picture or tell a story (spontaneous connected speech) and to raise his hand or in some way let the examiner know when he has produced an articulation error. This is typically the most difficult of the discrimination tests since consistently correct responses require that the child have a correct internal "image" of the target phoneme and an

ability to compare and contrast his own productions with that image. Generally, clients who are able to correctly identify their own errors without an external model but who, nonetheless, have articulation errors are thought to have phonetically-based defects. Such articulation disorders are normally due to neuromotor or structural defects. However, an exception may be found in the client who has received extensive auditory discrimination training in therapy but has not been given ample opportunity for phonetic production practice.

By testing a client's speech discrimination skills using the above three formats it is possible for the clinician to obtain a rather complete picture of any difficulty that might exist. By differentially identifying the level of the deficit, the clinician may more appropriately design and implement therapy strategies.

SEVERITY AND PROGNOSTIC DECISION MAKING

Factors affecting the clinician's estimate of severity and prognosis have been mentioned throughout the text. Such information is important to clinical decision making and will be summarized here. Speech pathologists faced with potentially large caseloads or waiting lists and the need to see clients on a priority basis will find the following information useful in making decisions. In addition, many children with articulation errors do not require speech therapy since their errors will prove to be self-correcting. While additional research is needed in this respect, there is sufficient evidence available to allow the clinician to make a reasonable prediction. Such decisions, however, should not be based on single factors but rather on multiple indicators. The prognostic value of each of the variables below is discussed.

1. *Age* may be an important variable when considering the expected age of developmental mastery of the phonemes of English, as presented in Chapter 3. By referring to Table IV the clinician may determine the ages at which 50 and 90 percent of children, respectively, master the individual phonemes. Some misarticulations may be age-appropriate. Children who are past the age at which 90 percent of the children have mastered a given phoneme will, in all likelihood, require therapy for the correction of the defective sound. In addition, errors with

phonemes that are normally mastered earlier in the developmental sequence constitute a more severe disorder.

2. *Phoneme Errors* are important in the severity-prognostic decision-making process. The larger the number of errors, the more severe the defect. As a general rule, children with more than four different sound errors at the kindergarten age will continúe to have difficulty at the age of eight or nine unless therapy is initiated. Error type may also contribute information. Omissions are considered more severe than substitutions and the latter more severe than distortions. However, an exception may be noted when the distortions are not close approximations of the target phonemes or when they reflect a neuromotor or structural defect. Vowel errors are more severe than consonant misarticulations, as a general rule, unless such errors reflect a dialectal variation. The frequency of occurrence of the defective phonemes in the language is also a consideration. Errors with frequently occurring phonemes constitute a more severe defect since intelligibility is more adversely affected.

3. *Feature Errors* per phoneme error should be considered. Age-appropriate phoneme errors typically involve only single distinctive feature errors. If all other variables are equal, defective sounds having multiple feature errors are more severe than single feature phoneme errors and the probability of spontaneous correction is less.

4. *Error Consistency* has been repeatedly demonstrated to be a significant prognostic indicator. Children with highly inconsistent sound errors have a greater likelihood of outgrowing them than children who are highly consistent. Children who correctly articulate a sound in 70 to 75 percent of the contexts will probably not require therapy for correction of the phoneme. Although age and the specific phoneme must be considered, children who have error consistencies higher than approximately 70 percent will probably require therapy.

5. *Error Stimulability*, like consistency, is considered to be an important variable. The greater the child's stimulability, the less severe the error and the greater the likelihood that it will prove to be self-correcting. Children who are highly stimulable on all of their error sounds will probably not require speech therapy if all other indicators are favorable.

6. *Oral Form Discrimination* ability has been shown to be related to the severity of articulation disorders. Children with poor oral form discrimination ability will probably evidence more misarticulations and, in general, have a poorer prognosis for spontaneously outgrowing their errors.

7. *Diadochokinesis and Fine Motor Skills* should be evaluated and considered in arriving at a statement of severity and prognosis. It has been demonstrated that clients with poor fine motor skills who misarticulate sounds in kindergarten continue to evidence articulation difficulty in the third grade. Clients with significantly slow diadochokinetic syllable rates and poor articulatory control will typically evidence more severe impairments and their errors will prove to be more resistant to correction.

8. *Speech Sound Discrimination* test results should provide additional information. Clients with moderate and severe discrimination problems typically have more severe articulation defects. Children past the age of eight with such deficits are in need of specialized help. Such children frequently have associated difficulty with auditory memory and sequential activity and manifest problems in learning to read. These children may be considered to have a generalized auditory learning disability and will, undoubtedly, require speech therapy for remediation of their articulation defects.

To reiterate, decisions concerning severity and prognosis should be made on the basis of multiple indicators and not on the implication of a single variable. Caseload selection is an important consideration, especially to the clinician working in the schools. Indices of severity and prognosis should be useful in deciding which children to see for therapy and which ones to retest the following year. For example, children with only one or two phoneme errors who are highly inconsistent and stimulable have a reasonably good chance of spontaneously outgrowing their errors and might be put on a list to be reevaluated at the beginning of the next school year. Attention could then be paid to those with more severe defects who are less likely to show spontaneous improvement.

REFERENCES

Bateman, H.: *A Clinical Approach to Speech Anatomy and Physiology.* Springfield, Thomas, 1977.

Boone, D.: *The Voice and Voice Therapy.* Englewood Cliffs, P-H, 1977.

Darley, F., Aronson, A., and Brown, J.: *Motor Speech Disorders.* Philadelphia, Saunders, 1975.

Darley, F. and Spriestersbach, D.: *Diagnostic Methods in Speech Pathology.* New York, Har-Row, 1978.

DuBois, E. and Bernthal, J.: A Comparison of three methods for obtaining articulatory responses. *J Speech Hear Disord, 43:*295-305, 1978.

Faircloth, M. and Faircloth, M.: An analysis of the articulatory behavior of a speech defective child in connected speech and in isolated word responses. *J Speech Hear Disord, 25:*51-61, 1970.

Fletcher, S.: Time-by-count measurement of diadochokinetic syllable rate. *J Speech Hear Res, 15:*763-770, 1972.

Fox, D. and Johns, D.: Predicting velopharyngeal closure with a modified tongue anchor technique. *J Speech Hear Disord, 35:*248-251, 1970.

Hutchinson, B.: The validation of articulation tests. *J Comm Disord, 5:*80-85, 1972.

Ingram, D.: *Phonological Disability in Children.* New York, Elsevier, 1976.

Johnson, J.: Clinical validity of the Taub Oral Panendoscope. *Ohio J Speech Hear, 9:*97-105, 1974.

McDonald, E.: *Articulation Testing and Treatment: A Sensory Motor Approach.* Pittsburgh, Stanwix, 1964.

———: *Deep Test of Articulation.* Pittsburgh, Stanwix, 1964.

———: *Screening Deep Test of Articulation.* Pittsburgh, Stanwix, 1968.

McDonald, E. and McDonald, J.: *Norms for the Screening Deep Test of Articulation.* An unpublished report of a longitudinal study supported in part by an ESEA Title III Grant, 1974-1976.

McNutt, J.: Oral sensory and motor behaviors of children with /s/ or /r/ misarticulations. *J Speech Hear Res, 20:*694-703, 1977.

McReynolds, L.: Phonetic and phonemic analysis of misarticulations. In Bradford, L. (Ed.): *Communicative Disorders: An Audio Journal for Continuing Education.* New York, Grune, 1977.

McReynolds, L. and Engmann, D.: *Distinctive Feature Analysis of Misarticulations.* Baltimore, Univ Park, 1975.

McReynolds, L. and Huston, K.: A distinctive feature analysis of children's misarticulations. *J Speech Hear Disord, 36:*155-167, 1971.

Mullen, P. and Whitehead, R.: Stimulus picture identification in articulation testing. *J Speech Hear Disord, 42:*113-118, 1978.

Nation, J. and Aran, D.: *Diagnosis of Speech and Language Disorders.* St. Louis, Mosby, 1977.

Nicolosi, L., Harryman, E., and Kresheck, J.: *Terminology of Communication Disorders.* Baltimore, Williams & Wilkins, 1978.

Paynter, E. and Bumpas, T.: Imitative and spontaneous articulatory assessment of three-year-old children. *J Speech Hear Disord, 42:*119-125, 1977.

Pendergast, K., Dickey, S., Selmar, J., and Soder, A.: *Photo Articulation Test.* Danville, Interstate, 1969.

Perkins, W.: *Speech Pathology: An Applied Behavioral Science.* St. Louis, Mosby, 1972.

Powers, G.: Cinefluorographic investigation of articulatory movements of selected individuals with cleft palates. *J Speech Hear Res, 5:*59-69, 1962.
Shafer, W., Hine, M. and Levy, B.: *A Textbook of Oral Pathology.* Philadelphia, Saunders, 1974.
Singh, S.: *Distinctive Features: Theory and Validation.* Baltimore, Univ Park, 1976.
Spriestersbach, D., Moll, K., and Morris, H.: Subject classification and articulation of speakers with cleft palate. *J Speech Hear Res, 4:*362-372, 1961.
Standel, J., Gardner, J. and Hannah, E.: Distinctive feature analysis. In Hannah, E. (Ed.): *Applied Linguistic Analysis II.* Pacific Palisades, Sencom Associates, 1977.
Taub, S.: The Taub Oral Panendoscope: a new technique. *Cleft Palate J, 3:*328-246, 1966.
Turton, L.: Diagnostic implications of articulation testing. In Wolfe, W. and Goulding, D. (Eds.): *Articulation and Learning.* Springfield, Thomas, 1973.
Van Demark, D.: A factor analysis of the speech of children with cleft palates. *Cleft Palate J, 3:*159-170, 1966.
Walsh, H.: On certain practical inadequacies of distinctive feature systems. *J Speech Hear Disord, 39:*32-42, 1974.
Wepman, J.: *Auditory Discrimination Test.* Los Angeles, Western Psych, 1973.
Yoss, K. and Darley, F.: Developmental apraxia of speech in children with defective articulation. *J Speech Hear Res, 17:*399-416, 1974.

CHAPTER 6

Treatment

GENERAL CONSIDERATIONS

ARTICULATION THERAPY, like most other forms of speech therapy, may be considered as basically compensatory in nature. The majority of the clients with articulation defects have, for one reason or another, failed to acquire the requisite phonemic or phonetic skills naturally. Thus, regardless of the specific approach selected, therapy is basically designed to provide the client with a compensatory program of intensified, controlled instruction, stimulation, and feedback. It is through such special attention and emphasis that we hope to improve the client's speech.

In order to be maximally effective, the therapy program must be tailored to the individual client. If we use the same approach to treat all of our articulation impaired clients we will undoubtedly mistreat the majority. Through the information obtained in our assessment we should attempt to design a therapy regimen that is appropriate to the etiology and nature of the defect and the client's individual strengths and weaknesses.

We should initially make every effort to eliminate or reduce the magnitude of untoward conditions or defects that may prove deleterious to progress in therapy. For example, if the client has a hearing loss, the clinician should seek audiological consultation and consider amplification if appropriate. If a structural defect such as cleft palate or ankyloglossia exists, the clinician should initiate appropriate medical referral to determine the potential for structural improvement. If parental attitude or the home environment constitute a problem, we should plan for a number of parent counseling or advisement sessions, either as preliminary to direct therapy with the client or as an integral part of it.

While it is not always possible to modify existing conditions, we can usually assist the client by helping him to compensate for them. In the case of poor auditory or tactile-kinesthetic dis-

181

crimination, we may work directly on improving such skills or we may stress the alternate auditory, tactile, or visual characteristics in working toward correction of defective sounds. The emphasis here is on considering the individual's needs in designing therapy. Of course it should be remembered that the best plans, no matter how well conceived, may prove to be ineffective. The speech pathologist should continually assess the client's responsiveness and progress with respect to a given therapy strategy and should be sufficiently flexible to modify or change approaches as the need dictates. A good therapist is a good diagnostician.

Throughout the book the author has emphasized the distinction between phonetic and phonemic disorders of articulation. In the case of a *predominantly phonemic disorder* the primary problem lies in the cognitive-conceptual domain. The client's knowledge of the sound system is in some way deviant. He has either failed to acquire a given distinctive feature(s) or has not mastered a rule(s) governing the correct combination of features to form specific phonemes. In the case of a *predominantly phonetic disorder* the primary problem lies with the actual articulomotor production of speech. The client may have mastered the phonemic concepts of the sound system but is unable to achieve accurate phonetic realization. The treatment of these two broad disorder types should differ, if not in the generic approach selected at least in the goals established and the emphasis placed on certain aspects of training.

In working with predominantly phonemic disorders therapy should focus on developing a conceptual awareness of the defective feature or rule with a possible emphasis on discrimination training. While some time may be spent on production, this is usually done for the purpose of reinforcing a feature distinction. It is assumed that the client has the phonetic skills necessary to produce the target phoneme.

With phonetically based disorders, however, the emphasis is typically on articulomotor production. Therapy methods are designed to establish correct production of the defective sound(s). While some attention is typically paid to discrimination training, it is usually considered as preliminary to phonetic modification or correction procedures. It is assumed that the child has an accurate concept of the target phoneme and that the primary difficulty lies with phonetic execution. The primary purpose of discrimination training with such a client is to make him aware that his phonetic production is not congruent with his phonemic concept and to develop a perceptual sensitivity to phonetic variations.

Of the major published approaches for the treatment of articulation disorders, some are best applied to phonetically based disorders while others are more applicable to phonemic disorders. Still others may be considered as somewhat generic in nature, having components applicable to the treatment of either disorder type. As each major approach is described its applicability will be discussed.

THE TRADITIONAL APPROACH

Van Riper and Irwin (1958), as discussed in Chapter 2, conceive of the traditional approach to the treatment of articulation disorders as based on servosystem or feedback theory. As the reader may recall from previous discussion, the developing child initially establishes an "auditory image" of the phonemes of his language through repeated exposure. The "image" may undergo some revision as the child becomes auditorily aware of (learns to discriminate) all of the features comprising a given phoneme. During this process, via feedback and self-monitoring, the child begins to establish a correspondence between his own articulatory output and his auditory image of the phoneme.

Through trial and error he may vary his output until he has established a subjective match. During this period the child monitors his outputs primarily via the auditory channel. At the same time, however, he establishes an association between his acoustic production and the kinesthetic information received from the articulators. At any rate, once the child believes that his output and auditory image are the same he will store the neuromotor commands associated with the kinesthetic and auditory feedback and will close the servosystem loop. As this occurs, the auditory channel typically looses monitoring primacy. The child's production becomes solidified and habituated. The established pattern of production becomes somewhat automatic, governed by a closed loop servosystem. Since the child believes that his auditory image of the phoneme is accurate and consistent with the external model provided by others, he stops listening critically to others' productions. Since he is comfortable with the perceived match between his production and his auditory image, he discontinues any effort to modify his pattern of production. Defective articulation may become stabilized in this manner.

Based on the above rationale, the first goal of therapy is to reopen the closed loop system. That is, the child with defective articulation must be encouraged to again listen critically to the speech of others and to revive his skills at self-hearing. According to the tenets of the traditional approach, this initial stage of therapy is necessary in order for the child to develop a correct auditory image of his defective phoneme(s), an awareness that his production(s) are inaccurate, and an ability to discriminate the nature of the difference between the target phoneme and his error production(s). Van Riper and Irwin refer to this stage of therapy as *ear training.*

While some clinicians have argued that ear training and the focus on developing auditory skills is unnecessary (See Perkins, 1971 for discussion), Van Riper and Irwin, as well as others, argue cogently that this stage of therapy is necessary and must be preliminary to work on production. Using servosystem theory as rationale, Van Riper suggests that the child must be taught to *scan* his own productions in terms of auditory and kinesthetic feedback and to *compare* his productions with that of the target phoneme before he can be expected to vary his phonetic output in the direction of the *correct* pattern. While not referring to a servosystem rationale, West, Ansberry and Carr (1937) advocate very similar goals for the initiation of therapy.

In his widely adopted 1972 text, Van Riper describes four techniques or steps of ear training and elaborates on each in order to provide the clinician with suggested activities attendant to each step. Briefly, Van Riper's suggested steps for ear training are as follows:

1. *Isolation,* in which the client is taught to focus on a target phoneme; to become aware of it in phonetic

contexts through a process of having the client listen to the sound as it is differentially emphasized through vocal intensity, prolongation and fragmentation; and to signal its presence whenever it occurs.

2. *Stimulation,* in which the client is auditorily "bombarded" and repeatedly exposed to the sound using amplification, a language master, tape recordings, etc., for the purpose of ensuring recognition and familiarity.
3. *Identification,* in which the client is taught to identify the salient characteristics of the target sound through a process of comparing and contrasting its auditory characteristics with those of other sounds.
4. *Discrimination,* the final step in which the client is taught to compare and contrast his error sound and the target sound, first as they are produced by others and then as they are produced by the client.

The second stage of therapy, *production training,* begins once the client is able to consistently identify his own productions as correct or incorrect in a variety of contexts. Work on correct production is done first at the level of the *isolated sound.* Once correct production is established at this level, the clinician then moves to work at the *syllable level.* As success is achieved with the sound in syllables, sound production in *words* and, finally, in *sentences* is systematically introduced. At each level above the isolated sound, work on establishing correct production of the target phoneme in a number of phonetic environments and in different positions, e. g. initial, medial, and final positions of words, is stressed. At each level the client is asked to scan, compare, vary, and correct his productions. Once established, activity designed to stabilize the newly learned pattern of production is introduced.

Van Riper describes five techniques that may be used to establish a target sound in production training. The first, *progressive approximation,* involves taking the client through a series of transitional sounds or phonetic postures, each being a closer approximation of the target sound, until the target sound is achieved. Typically, the clinician will begin by making the same error that the client makes and then, in small steps, will have the client imitate the successive approximations. As the client achieves success at each step he is rewarded. This technique is essentially the same as the operant procedure of "shaping," which involves the modification of behavior in small planned steps, selectively reinforcing target behaviors at each step.

The second technique, *auditory stimulation,* involves having the clinician simply model the target phoneme in isolation in an attempt to evoke a correct production by the client. Different auditory stimulation approaches, such as prolongation, stress, or amplification, may be tried.

A third technique, *phonetic placement,* is probably the single most widely used method. With this technique, the clinician typically provides the client with phonetic instruction concerning the placement of the articulators needed for correct production. The clinician may directly manipulate the client's articulators, with the aid of a tongue blade, to the correct positions or may provide the client with a phonetic model through the use of a mirror or diagram. The technique is an old one and may be found as a part of the early approaches conceived by Scripture in 1927 and Stinchfield-Hawk and Young in 1938 (Sommers, 1974).

A fourth technique, *modification of other sounds already mastered,* is somewhat like the progressive approximation technique described above. However, rather than moving in successive small steps, the client is asked to move from a sound he can produce to the target sound in one step. The clinician has the client produce and hold a sound he has already mastered. He is then instructed to move his articulators in a definite manner while continuing his production. The change is designed to produce an approximation of the target phoneme. The clinician may model the desired movement pattern before having the client attempt it. As an example, a client with a defective /s/ may be asked to produce the voiceless /th/ sound and to hold it briefly. From this position, he can be instructed to pull his tongue back slowly and to raise it behind his upper teeth as he continues the production. The new positioning should result in an approximation of the /s/ phoneme. Once the basic posturing is obtained, the clinician may have the client vary the placement slightly in order to obtain an accurate production.

The fifth technique Van Riper suggests is known as the *key word method*. With clients who are able to produce the target sound correctly in some phonetic contexts, words may be found in which correct production occurs. These words, key words, are then used as reference sources in which the clinician can emphasize correct production of the target sound. By having the client produce the key words and prolong or stress the target sound, the nature of its correct production can be emphasized and reinforced.

The third stage or goal in Van Riper's traditional approach involves *stabilization,* some clinicians refer to this as *habituation* and *carry-over*. This aspect of therapy focuses on achieving automatization of the correct production across phonetic and linguistic contexts and in all speaking situations or environments. Van Riper (1972) states that "essentially what we mean by stabilization is the maintaining of a target relationship under changing conditions." Until the target phoneme is consistently produced correctly in spontaneous connected speech under all speaking conditions and comes under automatic, closed loop control, we cannot consider the correction process complete.

Stabilization and carry-over training should not be viewed as a process completely separate from production training, beginning only after the latter is complete. For example, Van Riper suggests that we work on stabilizing or strengthening correct production of the target phoneme at each of the levels of isolation, syllable, word, and sentence before progressing to the next. Similarly, he suggests that we attempt to get carry-over of correct production outside of the therapy room by making home assignments relative to each level of production training. Of course, the final objective is to achieve stabilization and carry-over at the level of spontaneous connected speech. In both his 1958 and 1972 texts, Van Riper provides suggestions for strengthening correct productions at each level and for establishing carry-over. A few of these are discussed below.

One procedure for strengthening and stabilizing correct production involves having the client prolong, intensify, and exaggerate the sound while paying attention to the tactile and kinesthetic feedback associated with the correct production. The clinician may ask the client to feel the position and movements of his tongue, lips, etc., in order to heighten his haptic awareness of the sound. Some clinicians have employed auditory masking techniques in order to reduce or eliminate the auditory channel and force the client to monitor his productions via the tactile and kinesthetic feedback modalities. In the author's opinion this is a sound technique (excuse the pun) since preliminary research findings would tend to suggest that automatization of correct production requires a certain degree of reliance on tactile-kinesthetic monitoring (Manning et al., 1977).

Another suggested way to strengthen the target phoneme is to combine production with graphics. That is, the client is asked to prolong and exaggerate the sound and, at the same time, to write the letter. This should function to strengthen the association between correct production and the target phoneme.

Since articulation is, in part, a motor process, having the client produce the correct sound rapidly over a number of trials may help the pattern to become more automatic. This activity may also be done having the client alternately produce the target sound and other sounds in order to solidify the movement patterns involved in basic transitions.

Another technique, *negative practice,* involves having the client intentionally misarticulate the sound, using his error pattern, for the purpose of comparing the error with correct production and reinforcing or solidifying the critical distinctions.

Suggestions for achieving carry-over include an assortment of activities designed to elicit conversational speech under a variety of conditions, role playing and home assignments.

It should be obvious, even in light of the cursory review given above, that Van Riper's approach is a fairly comprehensive one. It provides the clinician with a definite rationale on which to base the suggested activities. The proposed procedures cover the entire spectrum from establishing awareness through achieving habituation. While Van Riper advocates following the suggested steps or proposed chronology for most clients, he also acknowledges that "there are many roads to Rome, many paths to success in articulation therapy" and suggests that it may be beneficial, for example, to begin therapy at the syllable or word level for some clients. The comprehensiveness of the approach makes it broadly applicable to a large variety of cases and the reader is encouraged not to think of the proposed steps or stages as inviolable. Adaptations of the suggested procedures to meet the needs of a given client would seem to be most appropriate and, in fact, should be encouraged.

The traditional approach might be considered as a generic one relative to its application to phonetic or phonemic disorders. Although its focus on production training at various levels would seem to make it more applicable to phonetically-based problems, the techniques that place emphasis on establishing a discriminative auditory awareness of the target phoneme would certainly be appropriate to the treatment of phonemic disorders. Again, because of its comprehensiveness and multiple components it may be applied to either disorder classification by emphasizing different aspects. This should not be interpreted by the reader as suggesting that, even with modification, it is always the preferred or most efficient approach to treating articulation disorders. Its merit lies in the wealth of suggested activities and its broad applicability.

THE SENSORIMOTOR APPROACH

Unlike the traditional approach's primary emphasis on auditory feedback and the acoustic nature of the target phoneme, the primary emphasis in sensorimotor therapy is on establishing the correct tactile and kinesthetic images associated with accurate production. The focus is almost exclusively on production training and is therefore most applicable to phonetically based disorders.

The primary proponent of sensorimotor therapy is Eugene McDonald. His text, *Articulation Testing and Treatment: A Sensory-Motor Approach,* published in 1964 has been widely adopted as the principle reference source for the approach. It provides both rationale and didactic instruction for the conduct of therapy.

McDonald suggests that the syllable is the basic unit of speech production and that articulation is a dynamic, ongoing process that consists of a "series of overlapping ballistic movements."

Thus, he does not believe that work at the level of the isolated sound and on static place of articulation postures is of much value. Rather, he stresses the need to work on defective sounds in syllables and phonetic contexts in order to emphasize the movement patterns associated with correct production. Therapy involves working on the defective sound in syllables, phonetic contexts of increasing complexity and finally in sentences. The primary purpose of McDonald's sensorimotor approach is to heighten the client's awareness of the tactile and kinesthestic patterns associated with correct production of the sound in identified facilitory contexts (see Chapter 5) and then to systematically increase the number of contexts in which the client can correctly produce the error sound.

In reviewing McDonald's proposed regimen, at least three phases of therapy are discernible. The first phase is designed to heighten a child's haptic awareness of the overlapping movements of articulation in general. It does not involve direct work on the client's error sound per se, but rather, is preliminary to it and designed to tune the client into the "feel" of articulatory movement patterns. As with all phases of therapy, an imitative stimulus-response approach is employed, i.e. the clinician provides an auditory model of the selected syllable combination and the client imitates the production. Following each production, the client is asked to describe the articulators involved in production, their direction of movement, points of contact, etc., with the help of the clinician. For example, the clinician may ask questions: (1) What did you feel when you said that? (2) Where did the tongue, lips, etc., touch? (3) Did the tongue move forward or backward in your mouth? (4) Where did the air go? (5) Did you make the sound in the front, middle, or back of your mouth?

During this phase, syllable combinations are selected that progress from simple to complex movement requirements. For instance, with a young child the clinician may choose to begin with a bisyllable such as /bibi/ placing equal stress on both syllables. In order to provide adequate practice and experience at this level of movement complexity, the clinician may select additional vowels (baba, bubu) and then additional consonants (didi, kuku) for drill.

McDonald suggests that the next step would involve differentially stressing the first and second bisyllables. Suggested progression from here would include the introduction of different vowels (bibu), different consonants (daga), different consonants and vowels (diga), and, finally, trisyllables such as /patiku/. Again, the progression is from simple to complex movement patterns and McDonald suggests that clinicians use their own discretion in selecting syllable drill material for the client. Only phonemes that the client is able to correctly produce should be used in this phase of therapy. In selecting the syllable combinations and progressions, the clinician should make certain that the place of articulation characteristics are sufficiently variable to provide a variety of sensorimotor patterns and that the required movements progress from large shifts to more subtle close proximity movements.

Phase two of McDonald's approach centers on the client's error sound and has the purpose of establishing and strengthening the sensorimotor patterns associated with correct production. This phase of therapy is initiated by selecting a phonetic context in which the client correctly articulates the error sound. As discussed in Chapter 5, such facilitory contexts may be identified through administration of McDonald's Deep Test of Articulation. Using the facilitory context, the clinician models the syllable (or word) combination, exaggerating each sound in the sequence using a slow motion production in order to emphasize the movement pattern. The client then imitates the production and, as in phase one, describes the articulatory movements and oral sensations associated with correct production. The process is repeated with varying stress on the two bisyllables. Then by using a picture (if two meaningful words are used) or a written presentation, the clinician may cover one word or a portion of one syllable and ask the client to prolong the target sound until the rest of the sequence is uncovered.

This process further emphasizes the correct sensorimotor feedback. With each activity the client is given ample opportunity for practice at the discretion of the clinician. The word or syllable combination(s) is then presented in a short sentence. The sentence does not have to make sense and the client is encouraged to suggest his own drill material. The sentences may be presented using a variety of stress patterns and, again, the client is asked to continue describing the sensorimotor patterns involved. Once the clinician believes that the tactile-kinesthetic images associated with the correct production of the target sound in a given context have been firmly established, the third phase of therapy is begun.

The third phase of McDonald's therapy regimen is designed to systematically increase the number of phonetic contexts in which the client correctly articulates the target sound. This phase may be initiated by first changing the vowel(s) used in the facilitory context in phase two. A vowel that is physiologically similiar to the one used in phase two may be selected if no other is identified through deep testing. Many of the steps in phase two may then be repeated. As the number of facilitating contexts increase, appropriate drill material may be added to a practice notebook that the client may use outside of the therapy session.

It is reasonable to assume that as the sensorimotor pattern associated with correct production becomes strengthened, additional facilitory contexts will appear and periodic deep testing for the purpose of identifying new contexts and checking progress in therapy is recommended. The third phase of therapy should continue through selecting other abutting consonants for drill. As with the selection of vowels, if another consonant cannot be found that is facilitory under deep testing, a consonant that has similar phonetic features to the original context(s) should be tried. As with phase two, drill includes varying stress, rate of production, prolonging the sound in a variety of contexts, and moving from bisyllable to sentence productions. Specific activities for habituation and carry-over outside of the therapy situation and the selection of appropriate material is left to the discretion of the clinician and the client.

McDonald's approach is in essence a form of *stimulus generalization training.* As stated above, therapy on the error sound is initiated by selecting a stimulus condition (phonetic context) in which the client can correctly articulate the sound and then involves a rather exacting process designed to systematically increase or generalize that response to other stimulus conditions (phonetic contexts). As noted earlier, it is an approach almost exclusively applicable to phonetic disorders. Unfortunately, many clients with such disorders are not inconsistent in their misarticulations. That is, many of these clients will be completely consistent in misarticulating an error sound. In such cases, deep testing will fail to reveal a facilitory context and, of course, you cannot generalize a response that does not exist. McDonald's approach does not provide for establishing a correct production. Thus, in order to apply this method with a client who is completely consistent in his error productions it would first be necessary to establish correct production and at least one facilitory context through other methods.

Despite its limitations, however, the approach may be beneficially applied to certain clients, possibly in adjunct with other methods. Once a target sound is established, sensorimotor therapy offers an efficient, systematic approach to generalization training. It would appear to be most applicable to clients with phonetically based disorders who, in light of the rather exacting participation requirements, are six or seven years of age or older.

THE DISTINCTIVE FEATURE APPROACH

Distinctive feature therapy may represent the most efficient approach to the treatment of phonemically based articulation disorders. As observed by McReynolds and Huston (1971), children are consistent in their feature errors and a few feature errors may account for many phoneme errors. For example, all of the fricative phonemes would be misarticulated by a child who has not mastered the single feature concept of plus frication. It would seem far more reasonable and efficient to work on developing the concept of frication than to work on each of the ten fricative phonemes separately. Research demonstrates that once a feature has been mastered in one or two representative error phonemes generalization across phonemes occurs to a significant extent. That is, the clinician only has to develop the feature concept in a few phonemes in order to correct the majority of phonemes defective because of the missing target feature (McReynolds and Bennett, 1972; Costello and Onstine, 1976).

Although distinctive feature theory has been well developed, clinical applications in the form of suggested therapy regimens have been slow in coming and a number of questions relative to the most efficient techniques remain unanswered. In 1970, Weber suggested that a feature concept may be developed by teaching a client to auditorily discriminate between contrastive, minimal phonemic pairs. In other words, by teaching a client to discriminate between two phonemes that differ only by one feature, the feature will become conceptually real to the client. Weber suggests that the error feature be trained in such a manner. For example, if a client substitutes /t/ for /s/, working with the client toward developing an ability to discriminate between the two phonemes should help him master the concept of frication, the only feature that makes the two phonemes distinctive.

McReynolds and Bennett (1972) were the first to report the results of a distinctive feature approach. Using Chomsky and Halle's Distinctive Feature System (see Chapter 1) they analyzed the articulation errors of three children and selected a target feature on which to train each child. In each case a phoneme containing the positive attribute of the feature was selected, together with a minimally contrastive phoneme that differed only in reference to the target feature.

Using a four-step program, they taught each child to differentially produce the contrastive phonemes, first in the initial position of a nonsense syllable and then in the final position. They employed an imitation response paradigm and incorporated principles of operant conditioning. The first step involved teaching the client to produce the phoneme containing the positive attribute of the target feature. The second step involved having the child produce the principle phoneme and the contrastive phoneme in a differential discriminative manner. Since an imitative response paradigm was employed, it forced the child to discriminate between the two phonemes, as auditorily modelled by the clinician, on the basis of the feature difference. McReynolds and Bennett report that feature errors were decreased by 69 to 84 percent and that error phonemes not worked on showed spontaneous correction, i.e. across phoneme generalization occurred as a result of the training program.

Costello and Onstine (1976) describe a feature therapy program that differed somewhat from the one described above. Rather than selecting only one defective phoneme that lacked the target feature, as McReynolds and Bennett suggest, they selected two and contrasted them both with the substitute phoneme. In the clients reported, the error phonemes /θ/ and /s/ were contrasted with the substitute phoneme /t/ in order to develop the feature of plus continuant. Two phonemes were used based on the rationale that it might be more effective in promoting across phoneme generalization. A second difference was that Costello and Onstine worked on establishing correct discriminative production at the levels of isolation, nonsense syllables, words, phrases, and sentences and, finally in conversational speech. A programmed approach was followed and principles of operant conditioning were employed.

Their reported results are quite impressive. One client required sixteen hours of therapy and the other twenty-five hours in order to achieve a criterion of 90 percent correct production of the two error phonemes at the level of conversational speech. Furthermore, spontaneous correction or improvement occurred on error phonemes not included in the therapy program. They state that "essentially seven error phonemes were changed as a function of instruction on three phonemes."

While it appears that distinctive feature therapy may be a highly efficient approach to the treatment of phonemic articulation disorders, there are at present more questions than answers concerning the format that should be followed. As Costello and Onstine suggest, there are several issues that need to be examined. For example, in the Costello-Onstine approach, the clients were taught to both produce two of their error sounds across phonetic contexts, being provided with ample opportunity for motor production practice, and, at the same time, were involved in learning the feature contrast.

Which aspect of therapy was responsible for the apparent success, the motor learning or the conceptual contrastive awareness of the feature? Are both aspects of therapy necessary or will only one suffice? What is the nature of the across phoneme generalization process? How is it that other phonemes, which are defective because of a missing feature, show spontaneous correction when the child acquires the feature in another phoneme? Does the client in some way realize that the newly acquired feature is the element that has been missing from his other defective phonemes? Does this mean that he must be aware that the other phonemes are defective? Is some motor production practice needed once the client has acquired the feature concept in order to establish it within his production repertoire? These are difficult questions and as of this writing are unanswered. Until they are we will have to continue with our experimental therapy strategies.

Interestingly, both of the clients used by Costello and Onstine had partially developed the feature of continuancy since it was reported that they correctly produced the phonemes /f/ and /v/. Thus, the feature was already in their conceptual and production repertoires. It might have been enlightening had they selected the /f/ and /v/ and contrasted them with the /p/ and /b/ phonemes, respectively, in order to reinforce the concept of the continuancy feature. The results of such an approach might have at least partially answered some of the above questions. Further, it is possible that a strict auditory discrimination approach that first emphasized the /p/-/f/ and /b/-/v/ contrasts and then incorporated a few of the error phoneme contrasts such as /t/-/s/ might have proven effective in obtaining the same results reported above. However, for the time being this must be considered purely speculative since differential efficacy studies have not been reported.

As the reader may have guessed by now, the actual techniques employed in distinctive feature therapy do not differ from other approaches already discussed. What makes it different from other approaches is the selection of stimulus material (based on the distinctive feature analysis), the use of paired contrasts and the focus on feature concept development. Whether or not an auditory discrimination paradigm alone is sufficient to fully develop the feature concept and achieve correct articulation of the target phonemes is unknown. Distinctive feature therapy must be considered as still in the experimental stage of development; clinicians must rely on their own creative juices and clinical judgment in designing techniques of implementation.

The author's own bias is that some production training is probably necessary in order to obtain complete correction. This is based largely on the following assumptions: (1) feature concepts are comprised of both auditory-acoustic and articulomotor components; (2) differential production of the minimal pairs reinforces the feature concept; and, (3) consistency in the correct production of the feature requires some motor practice across a variety of phonetic contexts. It is also the author's belief that with clients who correctly articulate at least one phoneme containing the target feature (the majority do), discrimination concept training should be initiated with that phoneme. Since the target feature is already a part of the client's conceptual repertoire, it seems wasteful not to capitalize on it. Of course, it will probably still be necessary to incorporate some of the error phonemes into the process but the task should be made easier by first emphasizing the feature contrast using a phoneme the client has already mastered.

As an example of the above and to illustrate some of the techniques the author has used with some success, let us consider the hypothetical client discussed in Chapter 5. As the reader may recall, the client had the following substitution errors: t/s; d/z; t/ʃ; d/ʒ; p/f; and b/v. The feature analysis revealed that, in each case, the error involved substituting a plosive for a fricative. As discussed in Chapter 5, although place errors were noted in four of the sound substitutions they were considered as artifacts of the manner error. Therefore, the feature of plus frication should be selected as the target for therapy. Since the phonemes /θ/, /ð/, /h/ and /hw/ were all produced correctly, we may assume that the target feature is well within the client's conceptual repertoire. Therapy might then be initiated by selecting the /θ/-/t/ and /ð/-/d/ as reasonable contrastive pairs to begin training.

The first step would involve having the client listen to the clinician produce slightly prolonged or emphasized versions of the phoneme pairs. After each pair the clinician may ask the client to identify the elements as same or different. Since it is assumed that the client will be able to recognize that they are indeed different, he will then be asked to describe the nature of the difference. The clinician may help by asking such questions as "is the first one longer or shorter than the second one?"

The concept might be further developed by having the client move his finger along the table top as long as the phoneme is being produced, emphasizing the fact that the fricative phoneme is continuous while the plosive is abrupt and not continuous. The phoneme pairs may then be presented in minimal word pairs and, finally in phrases containing the word pairs. At each level the discrimination task is continued with the client reinforced for his correct judgments.

Step two involves selecting one or two of the error phonemes to be added to one of the above target phonemes. Since the substitute phoneme for both /s/ and /ʃ/ is the same, /t/, these might be selected, along with /θ/ above to be contrasted with /t/. Step one would then be repeated using the contrastive pairs, /θ/-/t/, /s/-/t/. In all three pairs the feature of plus frication is emphasized and, since it has already been trained in the /θ/-/t/ pair, generalization to the error phonemes /s/ and /ʃ/ should be accomplished rather easily.

Step three involves both production and discrimination. Once the client has demonstrated a high level of accuracy in step two (say 90% correct discrimination), the clinician should then model one of the elements of each pair, sometimes the target phoneme and sometimes the replacement phoneme /t/, and ask the client to produce it. The client is then asked if his production is the same as that of the clinician. The client is rewarded for correct judgments. In this manner, the discrimination paradigm is continued but with the addition of production practice and the requirement to compare his own production with an external source.

For some clients it may be necessary to provide some phonetic instruction concerning the production of the feature in the error phonemes. However, this requirement, if it occurs, should re-quire little effort since the feature is already produced correctly in one of the elements, /θ/. As the client achieves success at the level of the isolated phonemes, the paradigm is systematically continued through minimal pair words and phrases. Once the client is able to differentially produce the three phonemes paired at the level of minimal pair words in phrases and is able to accurately compare his productions with those of the clinician, step four may be initiated.

The initiation of step four assumes that the client has obtained an auditory-acoustic and articulomotor concept of the fricative feature in both the error phonemes /s/ and /ʃ/. It involves so-lidifying the concept via self-monitoring. The client is asked to produce the target phonemes without an auditory model from the clinician and to make judgments of correct or incorrect. The client's correct judgments are reinforced and as success is achieved at the level of the isolated phoneme, the clinician systematically presents material at the word, phrase, and, eventually, conversational speech level. At the end of step four, the clinician should retest the error phonemes to determine the extent of generalization. It is sometimes necessary to select one or two additional error phonemes, which do not evidence spontaneous correction, for additional training.

The four steps above reflect the author's own experimental strategy in employing distinctive feature theory in the therapy room. While it has proven successful for many clients, it has been necessary to modify it with others. It is offered to the reader only as one example; modifications for clinical trial are encouraged. For example, the clinician may wish to subject error phonemes to deep testing in order to design contextual stimulus material for use in steps three and four. It should be obvious that the author has simply modified traditional therapy techniques and incorporated them into a distinctive feature framework.

Distinctive feature therapy offers great promise as an extremely efficient mode for the treatment of phonemic articulation disorders. To reiterate, focus on the single dimension of the phonemes in error and the ability to work on several defective phonemes at once should prove a significant savings of time in the correction process. The selection of representative phonemes for feature training should maximize the generalization process. While generalization is still not completely understood, Sommers (1974) states that "it seems logical that distinctive feature clusters for each phoneme have corollary clusters of sensory and motor feedback networks in all modalities . . . so that emphasis on a feature from a distinctive feature cluster should produce a perceptual and motor learning which fosters and maximizes sound generalization."

MINIMAL CONTRAST THERAPY

In working with phonemically based articulation disorders, it is not uncommon to find that you are able to establish correct production of a target sound in isolation and at the level of the nonsense syllable but not in meaningful words. Resistance to correct production at the word level often proves to be frustrating for the clinician and client alike. Undoubtedly it is at least partially attributable to prior learning and the strong associations that have been established between semantic referents and verbal utterances. For example, to a child with a t/s error the yellow ball that appears in the daytime sky may indeed be a "tun." The semantic association will frequently interfere with the client incorporating the newly acquired /s/ into the word "sun" or other verbal constructs in which the t/s has been solidified and signifies meaning.

An approach that the author has found to be quite useful with such clients is Cooper's (1968) Minimal Contrast Therapy. The approach is designed to break up the semantic association between the referent and the defective verbal utterance and replace it with the correct verbal production. The technique involves creating an imaginary referent for the defective utterance and contrasting the pairing with the accurate production-original referent pair in order to force the distinction.

To illustrate the process we can use the above example of a child who substitutes t/s and says "tun" for "sun." The clinician first selects two pictures for presentation, one picture of the sun and the other a nonsense picture (may be drawn) to be paired with "tun." The clinician presents both pictures and labels them, i.e. this is "tun" and this is "sun." The clinician then has the client point to each picture after he names it and rewards correct identifications.

Once the client is able to differentially identify the two pictures without error, the clinician then establishes the functions of the two objects, i.e. this is the sun, it shines brightly in the sky in the day time, etc., and this is a "tun," you can play with it, throw it in the air, toss it to a friend, etc. The clinician then names the pictures, one at a time, and asks the child to explain their different functions. This activity is designed to establish the differential association between the two utterances and the two different referents and is continued until the client shows a complete understanding of the different functions. The child is rewarded for correct responses.

The third stage of therapy involves working on differential production. Since the client is able to discriminate between the two sounds (words) and is able to produce the target /s/ in isolation and nonsense syllables, differential production should not be difficult to obtain in light of the newly trained semantic referents. In this stage of therapy, the clinician points to one of the pictures, names it and then asks the child to describe its function and then to name it. The clinician is free to use any techniques that might be helpful in eliciting correct, differential productions.

Once the child is able to differentially produce the two words, another word pair involving the t/s contrast is selected and the process is repeated. Although not stated by Cooper, it is assumed that the selection of additional minimal pairs for contrast training should continue until generalization occurs and the child is correctly producing the target phoneme at the word level. However, it has been the author's experience that once one or two correct word productions are established, it is only necessary to use an imitative naming approach with a list of words containing the target sound (including the originally trained words and reinforcement for correct productions) to obtain generalization.

It should be mentioned that Cooper did not design his approach solely for the purpose of working with clients who have difficulty at the word level. However, the author feels that it is probably best suited for such special purpose and that it is probably inadequate as a major or sole approach to the treatment of articulation defects. It would certainly not be beneficial for all clients and might constitute a waste of time for clients who do not evidence difficulty moving from isolation or syllable to meaningful words. It does, however, represent an excellent strategy for younger children manifesting difficulty in this respect.

THE PAIRED STIMULI TECHNIQUE

The Paired Stimuli Technique, developed by Weston and Irwin (1971), has been shown to be an effective approach to phoneme generalization training. According to Irwin and Griffith (1973), it is an efficient method especially suitable for use in the school setting. Procedures are highly structured and based on principles of operant conditioning. The technique is applicable to clients with articulation disorders who have some spontaneous speech and are able to correctly articulate a given target sound in at least one word. The only materials required are pictures that depict words containing the target sound in the initial *or* final position and tokens (poker chips) for reinforcement of socially acceptable productions. Clinicians may develop their own materials or may purchase a commercially available *Paired Stimuli Kit.*

Fundamentally, the approach is one of stimulus generalization training. For clients able to correctly articulate a sound in one stimulus context (word), the approach is designed to increase the number of stimulus contexts (different words) in which the sound is correctly produced. For clients who are 100 percent consistent in their errors it would be necessary to first use other approaches in order to establish a given target sound in at least one context (word) prior to employing the Paired Stimuli Technique.

The first step involves the selection of *key* and *training* words. All words selected must contain the target sound only once, appearing in either the initial or final position. *Training words,* by definition, are those in which the client misarticulates the target sound at least two out of three times. The procedure for selecting training words involves having the client name ten or more pictures of words containing the sound in the initial position and ten or more pictures with the sound in the final position. The naming trials are repeated three times. Any word in which the target sound is misarticulated two times or more during the three trials may be selected as a training word. Pictures may be added until a total of ten training words with the sound in the initial position and ten training words with the sound in the final position have been selected. It is possible that some clients may need to work only on the sound in one position, i.e., fewer than ten training words may be found containing the target sound in a given position.

Key words are those in which the client correctly articulates the target sound, in either the initial or final position, at least nine out of ten times. Potential key words may be located during the selection of training words. Any word in which the sound is correctly articulated two or three times may be selected for naming an additional seven times. Although the reader may wonder about the necessity of having the client name a potential key word ten times, it is important that the context (word) be highly stable and that the client be able to consistently produce the sound correctly in the key word. If a key word cannot be located, one may be established by traditional methods, or the clinician may follow guidelines suggested by Irwin and Weston (1971).

Once a key word and ten training words containing the phoneme in a given position (initial or final) have been selected, training may start. The pictures of the ten training words are placed around the key word picture. The client is asked to alternately name key word and each of the ten training words. Each correct production of the target phoneme is rewarded with a token, whether produced in the key word or one of the training words. Incorrect productions are ignored, i.e. not rewarded. Accumulated tokens may be exchanged at the end of each therapy session for primary reinforcers, such as candy, toys, etc.

The repeated pairing of the reinforced correct production in the key word with each of the training words should result in generalization over repeated trials. Weston and Irwin suggest that the pairing of the key word with each of the ten training words constitutes a *training string* and that each training session should consist of three training strings. They also suggest that the clinician should keep a record of the number of correct productions in each training string and should administer pre- and posttraining session probes in order to determine the extent of generalization.

The presession and postsession probes consist of having the client name the key word and each of the ten training words (all twenty, if training words for both positions have been selected) without reinforcement. The suggested criterion for terminating training on a given phoneme in a given position is eight out of ten correct productions of the target phoneme in the ten training words on two successive post probes. Once the criterion is reached for the target sound in one position, work begins with the training words containing the phoneme in the opposite position. Once criterion is reached for both positions, a new target phoneme may be selected for training.

In describing the Paired Stimuli Technique, Irwin and Griffith (1973) state the following:

> Early in training, a child may earn few, if any, tokens for production of the target phoneme in training words because they are, by definition, phonetic environments in which he does not produce the target phoneme acceptably. However, he should produce the target phoneme in the key word acceptably at least nine out of ten times in each string. Otherwise, the key word is regarded as unstable and training must be temporarily discontinued, so that the key word may be brought to criterion again. With the continued contingent pairing of the key word and each training word, the child's correct production of the target phoneme in the key word begins to generalize to the training words, which are then also reinforced with tokens (p. 176).

A number of different training designs are described by Irwin and Weston (1971). They are primarily based on consideration of whether one or two key words are used in training and the position of the target phoneme in the key word(s). The interested reader is invited to consult the reference source.

The primary objective of generalization therapy is correct production of the target phoneme in spontaneous connected speech. Clinicians may, therefore, wish to extend paired stimuli training from the word level to phrases and sentences, varying the phonetic contexts in which the target sound appears and at the same time systematically fading the client's reliance on tangible reinforcements. With such extensions, the paired stimuli approach may be considered an extremely efficient method for generalization training. In light of its structure and efficiency with respect to time utilization, it would appear to be especially suitable for use in the school setting.

PARENT DIRECTED THERAPY

Under certain circumstances and with clients who evidence uncomplicated articulation defects, training parents to work with their own youngsters may represent a viable alternative to clinician directed approaches. If effective, such an approach would certainly be efficient in terms of allowing the speech pathologist to maximize his use of time. Time normally spent in the therapy room with such clients might be reallocated to clients with more difficult or complex defects. While more research is needed to determine the efficacy of parent administered approaches, a number of studies have already been reported (Sommers et al., 1959; Tufts and Holliday, 1959; Sommers, 1962; Sommers et al., 1964; Carrier, 1970; McCroskey and Baird, 1971; Shelton et al., 1978).

In 1959, Sommers et al. reported the results of what might be viewed as an intensive, structured parent education and home carry-over program. Parents participating in the program observed therapy sessions conducted by professionals, were provided with daily thirty minute lecture discussions on speech development and how to work with articulation defects and were instructed on how to work with their children at home. At the completion of the experimental program, the children who participated showed greater gains than a group of matched articulation defective children who received therapy without parent participation.

In the same year, Tufts and Holliday report a study in which thirty preschool-aged children with moderately severe articulation defects were randomly assigned to one of three groups. The first group did not receive therapy (maturational control group). The second group received traditional articulation therapy administered by professionals for a total of forty-six one-half hour sessions. The children in the third group received therapy administered by their parents. The parents met for one hour each week for twenty-five weeks and were given instruction on the fundamentals of traditional articulation therapy. Each session allowed question and answer periods in order to address specific problems. Tufts and Holliday report that at the end of the approximately seven month study, the children in groups two and three showed the same degree of improvement while those in group one did not improve. Although this study had some design limitations, e.g. the use of a rating scale as the criterion measure of improvement, the results are nonetheless interesting and support the efficacy of a parent directed approach.

A clinical study by Carrier (1970) is frequently cited as evidence for the support of parent directed approaches. Carrier's program employed an operant framework and involved teaching mothers how to present stimuli, evaluate responses, and apply consequences. Children with articulation disorders were first taught to correctly imitate a target sound by a professional clinician. The mothers were then taught how to elicit responses using picture cards that contained the target sound in the initial and final positions. The mothers worked with their children, reinforcing correct productions with verbal praise and tokens (the tokens, poker chips, could be exchanged for tangible rewards at the end of each session). Results revealed that all of the experimental subjects improved their articulation as a result of the parent administered program. Carrier also reports that sound generalization to conversational speech was beginning to occur for the children participating in the experimental program.

The total amount of time for the program was three weeks with only a one and one-half hours expenditure of professional time per child. Interestingly, the success of the program occurred "independent of such factors as educational levels and socioeconomic levels of the mothers." However, other studies have suggested that variables such as the intelligence of the child and maternal attitude are important in considering children for participation in parent directed approaches (Sommers, 1962; Sommers et al., 1964).

The following is intended as a general outline of goals and procedures that might prove to be effective in training parents to work with their articulatory defective children. As suggested by the screening criteria below, it is not intended for all clients. The criteria are designed for the purpose of selecting children who stand the greatest chance of being helped by such a program. The primary reason for employing a Parent Directed Program (PDP) is to save professional time. However, if a PDP requires more of the professional's time than directing the therapy himself then obviously the primary purpose is defeated. The selection criteria will hopefully avoid this. The PDP is offered to the reader for clinical trial and flexibility in dealing with particular parent-child problems is encouraged, i.e. it should not be considered as sacrosanct or inviolable.

Screening

It is felt that those parents and children meeting the following criteria will make the best candidates for the PDP. Much of the information may be obtained during the initial assessment and interview session(s).

The Child:
1. Should be relatively free of any clinically significant sensory, structural or neurological defects.
2. Should be between five and twelve years of age.
3. Should be at least 25 percent stimulable on his error sound(s).
4. Should be able to correctly produce the target sound(s) in some context, i.e. should not be 100 percent consistent in his error(s).
5. Should have no more than four separate phoneme errors.
6. Should have an intelligence capability within broad normal limits.

The Parent:
1. Should be free of speech, language, or hearing defects.
2. Should express a willingness to participate in the PDP once the responsibilities and nature of the Program have been explained.
3. Should manifest a positive rapport with the child and have a healthy attitude toward the child's speech defect.

Goals and Procedures

GOAL I: Provide the parent with a basic understanding of the processes of speech sound production and speech development, including the acquisition and mastery of articulation skills through feedback and principles of learning.

Procedures:
1. Discussion and descriptive techniques using appropriate models, charts, drawings, etc.

GOAL II: Familiarize the parent with the child's specific articulation error(s), their nature and related problems.

Procedures:
1. Describe the child's error(s) to parent.

2. Use a tape recorded sample of the child's speech and focus the parent's attention on the specific error(s).
3. Demonstrate the error(s) by having the child produce the target sound(s) in the parent's presence, pointing out the specific auditory and phonetic nature of the error(s).
4. Discuss and demonstrate any related or underlying deficits, e.g. poor auditory discrimination ability.

GOAL III: Provide the parent with an ability to consistently identify the occurrence of the child's error sound(s) and to consistently discriminate the error(s) and target sounds(s).

Procedures:
1. Have the parent listen to the child produce the target sound(s) and indicate whether each production is correct or in error:
   A. At the word level
   B. At the sentence level
   C. In spontaneous, connected speech.
2. Clinician will appropriately reinforce the parent's correct judgments.
3. If the parent has difficulty at level 1-A above, the clinician should demonstrate by having the child produce words containing the target sound(s) and indicating to the parent the accuracy of each production. Step 1-A should then be repeated. If still unsuccessful, go back to Goal II for additional training or terminate the PDP.

GOAL IV: Provide the parent with an understanding of how to work with the child on improving auditory discrimination of the error sound(s) and an ability to demonstrate the necessary procedures.

Procedures:
1. With the parent present, the clinician will work with the child and demonstrate having the child:
   a. Discriminate between correct and error productions of the target sound(s) when produced by the clinician.

b. Compare and contrast the accuracy or similarity of his own target sound production with those of the clinician.

The above should be conducted at the level of the isolated sound, and each step should be explained to the parent. Reinforcement procedures should be demonstrated.

2. Once some success has been obtained at the level of the isolated sound, the parent should demonstrate the above steps with the child at the word level. The clinician should provide the parent with appropriate instruction, feedback and reinforcement. Procedure number one may be repeated as needed to provide the parent with an understanding of technique.

Note: With the completion of Goal IV, the parent may, at the *discretion of the clinician* be assigned homework activity with the child and may be asked to review any or all of the preceding goals or procedures at the start of a given counseling therapy session to insure carry-over.

GOAL V: The parent will gain an understanding of generalization training and will be able to appropriately elicit, evaluate, and reinforce the child's correct productions of the target sound(s) as they occur in the initial and final positions of single words.

Procedures:
1. The clinician will select two or three key words in which the child has demonstrated an ability to produce the target sound correctly in the initial position and two or three key words with the sound in the final position. If there are no key words within the child's repertoire, the clinician will work with the child directly using appropriate phonetic procedures in order to establish key words.

2. The clinician will discuss and demonstrate the fact that the child can produce the target sound correctly in a few words but not the majority and that the object of future work is to increase the child's ability to produce the target sound(s) correctly in all contexts.

3. Using the key words, the clinician will demonstrate

how to elicit correct productions using picture presentations and how to reinforce correct responses with
a token system of reward.

4. The parent will then demonstrate procedure number
three with the child as the clinician observes and
makes suggestions.

5. The clinician will demonstrate eliciting word productions using non-key word picture presentations
coupled with auditory modelling in which the target
sound is stressed.

6. The parent will then demonstrate procedure number
five with the child and will reinforce correct productions and ignore incorrect responses.

7. The clinician will explain that once a high rate of
correct responses are elicited using procedure
number five the auditory modelling should be discon-
tinued.

8. The clinician will then select a number of key words
and non-key words for homework drill, with instructions to the parent that she should spend approximately one hour each day on the exercise and that as
success is obtained on the non-key words, other words
(pictures from magazines, etc.) may be selected for
drill. It should be explained that each drill session
must include some of the key words so that the correct
production can be reinforced.

GOAL VI: The parent will demonstrate an ability to monitor
the child's productions of the target sound(s) in connected
speech and to selectively reinforce correct productions.

Procedures:

1. The clinician will demonstrate having the child verbally describe pictures and selective reinforcement
techniques using both the token system and verbal
praise.

2. The parent will demonstrate procedure number one
with the child in the presence of the clinician.

3. The clinician will discuss the home program with the

parent and will make appointments for follow-up assessment to determine efficacy.

All of the goals, procedures and steps in the PDP, as outlined above, may not be necessary for all clients and may be modified for maximal efficiency. Much of the professional's time is normally spent with the client on discrimination and production generalization drills. For clients meeting the selection criteria, the potential savings in time should provide adequate impetus for clinical experimentation with the program. Furthermore, for many clients the higher degree of parental awareness and attention may result in a more effective effort than the traditional clinician-directed approaches.

THERAPEUTIC EFFICACY

Experimental evidence to support the assumption that one therapy method may be comparatively more effective than another for a given client is lacking. Undoubtedly, until such evidence is forthcoming, the choice of a given approach will continue to be based largely on each clinician's own bias and preference. Even if comparative efficacy could be established in a general sense, all clients, even those with similar disorders, are not equally responsive to a given therapy strategy. This means that in order to be effective, clinicians must master a number of different approaches for clinical trial. An effective clinician must have a number of techniques in his therapeutic armamentarium.

However, despite the lack of experimental evidence, the clinician may rely on clinical logic in the initial selection of a therapy method for a given client. With the presentation of each approach discussed here, the author has offered his own clinical insights concerning each method's applicability to phonetic and phonemically based articulation disorders. Further, the selection of a given approach should also include consideration of the client's particular needs and the therapeutic purpose. That is, the approaches differ in that some are designed to establish correct production while others focus on sound generalization or habituation training. Indeed, it is certainly possible to use a number of approaches with a given client relative to different stages of therapy, i.e. establishment, generalization, habituation, and carry-over.

In fact, a number of individuals have combined the basic facets of several of the approaches discussed here into an eclectic approach. An example may be found in the proposals by Winitz (1975). Winitz, in essense, developed a multifaceted approach that incorporates the concepts of progressive auditory discrimination training, conceptual training using minimal phoneme pairings, and production training using the principles inherent in sensorimotor therapy. Winitz suggests that the application of a given component, e.g. the need for discrimination or production training, should depend upon the individual client's needs. Such an approach might certainly prove effective with a large variety of clients, considering the differential applicability of its components. The creative clinician should be able to design similar eclectic approaches to meet the needs of any given client.

In addition to the question of the potential effectiveness of a given therapy approach, clinicians must also consider issues relative to scheduling. How often and for how long should the clinician see a client in order to be effective? Is group therapy as effective as individual therapy? These questions are of more than academic interest to practicing clinicians concerned with maximizing their use of time.

With reference to the first question, clinical experience would suggest that it is better to see a client for a number of short sessions each week than for one longer session. That is, if an option is available, the clinician should probably elect to see a client for two or three thirty-minute sessions each week rather than scheduling one long session of an hour or an hour and one-half duration. Of course the duration of each session should depend upon such factors as the age of the client, attention span, and tolerance level, in addition to considerations of time available. Under optimal conditions the client might be seen each day for a thirty minute or one hour session. However, this is hardly realistic for most clinicians regardless of work setting. The minimum amount of time that a clinician can schedule a client and still have a reasonable expectation for progress is somewhat uncertain and probably varies with each client. However, as a general rule of thumb, if a client cannot be seen for at least one intensive thirty minute session each week the clinician should seriously question the potential efficacy of therapy.

The question of the comparative efficacy of group and individual therapy is probably of greatest interest to clinicians working in the school setting. The issue has been investigated by Sommers (1962) and Sommers et al. (1966). In the latter study, seventeen clinicians worked with 240 mild and moderately articulation impaired children for eight and one-half months using traditional therapy methods. All of the children had normal hearing, were of normal intelligence, and apparently were free of any structural or neurological deficits. Half of the children received group therapy and half were scheduled to be seen individually. The results revealed the group and individual therapy to be equally effective in reducing articulation errors, regardless of the grade level of the children or their degree of articulation defectiveness. These results are impressive and should certainly reassure clinicians concerning the potential efficacy of group therapy.

Some deliberation should be given to the assignment of clients to groups. Sommers et al., for example, put mildly impaired youngsters in groups together and moderately impaired children together. Other factors that might be considered, relative to establishing reasonably homogeneous groups, include similar phoneme or feature errors and stimulability. For some clients who are free of structural or neurological problems, group therapy may actually have an advantage relative to the opportunity for vicarious learning.

Under conditions where it is necessary for the clinician to give priority to certain clients waiting for therapy, articulation defective individuals with high or moderate error consistency and moderate or low stimulability should be seen first. As referenced earlier in the book, individuals with low error consistency and high stimulability have a greater chance of spontaneously correcting their errors. Thus, maximum benefit from therapy will normally be achieved by those clients who are consistent in their errors and not very stimulable. These children usually do not improve significantly without therapeutic intervention and, therefore, have the greatest need. Caseload selection, in this respect, is another consideration in the clinician's effective use of time.

Regardless of the therapy approach selected, progress should be periodically assessed in order to determine efficacy. There are a number of ways to determine whether or not progress is being made. The clinician may periodically take a spontaneous speech sample and do a phonetic analysis, comparing the number of errors or contexts in which the error occurs with a sample taken previously. However, a more efficient and economical probe for progress might be to employ the McDonald Deep Test in order to ascertain the extent of generalization or to employ a standardized *Speech Production Task,* as conceived by Shelton, Elbert, and Ardnt (1967).

As previously mentioned, it is also possible to determine the degree of habituation by administering the sound production probe, whatever its nature, under conditions of masking. A solidified, stable production of a target phoneme should not break down under conditions of auditory masking. Of course, the probe used should be congruent with the specific objective(s) of a given stage of therapy and should be sufficiently sensitive to detect change or progress. The probe should be administered prior to beginning therapy and at various intervals during therapy in order to determine progress. Another way is to chart behaviors during each therapy session, that is, record and tally the total number of correct and incorrect responses during each session. However, many clinicians object to this procedure, suggesting that it interferes with rapport and therapeutic interaction. Regardless of the procedure selected, it is important for clinicians to establish indices of articulation change. Only by using such measures will they be able to ascertain the effectiveness of their strategies with clients and decide when modifications are needed.

REFERENCES

Carrier, J.: A program of articulation therapy administered by mothers. *J Speech Hear Disord, 35:*344-353, 1970.

Cooper, R.: The method of meaningful minimal contrasts in functional articulation problems. *J Speech Hear Assoc Va, 10:*17-22, 1968.

Costello, J. and Onstine, J.: The modification of multiple articulation errors based on distinctive feature theory. *J Speech Hear Disord, 41:*199-215, 1976.

Irwin, J. and Griffith, F.: A theoretical and operational analysis of the Paired Stimuli Technique. In Wolfe, W. and Goulding, D. (Eds.): *Articulation and Learning.* Springfield, Thomas, 1973.

Irwin, J. and Weston, A.: *A Manual for the Clinical Utilization of the Paired Stimuli Technique.* Memphis, Nat Ed Serv, 1971.

McCroskey, R. and Baird, V.: Parent education in a public school program of speech therapy. *J Speech Hear Disord, 36:*499-505, 1971.

McDonald, E.: *Articulation Testing and Treatment: A Sensory-Motor Approach.* Pittsburgh, Stanwix, 1964.

McReynolds, R. and Bennett, S.: Distinctive feature generalization in articulation training. *J Speech Hear Disord, 37:*462-470, 1972.

McReynolds, R. and Huston, K.: A distinctive feature analysis of children's misarticulations. *J Speech Hear Disord, 36:*155-166, 1971.

Manning, W., Wittstruck, M., Loyd, R., and Campbell, T.: Automatization of correct production at two levels of articulatory acquisition. *J Speech Hear Disord, 42:*358-363, 1977.

Perkins, W.: *Speech Pathology: An Applied Behavioral Science.* St. Louis, Mosby, 1971.

Shelton, R., Elbert, M., and Ardnt, W.: A task for evaluation of articulation change: II. Comparison of task scores during baseline and lesson series testing. *J Speech Hear Res, 10:*578-586, 1967.

Shelton, R., Johnson, A., and Ruscello, D.: Assessment of parent-administered listening training for preschool children with articulation deficits. *J Speech Hear Disord, 43:*242-254, 1978.

Sommers, R.: Factors in the effectiveness of mothers trained to aid in speech correction. *J Speech Hear Disord, 27:*178-186, 1962.

Sommers, R.: Nature and remediation of functional articulation disorders. In Dickson, S. (Ed.): *Communication Disorders: Remedial Principles and Practices.* Glenview, Scott, 1974.

Sommers, R., Furlong, A., Rhodes, F., Fichter, G., Bowser, D., Copetas, F., and Saunders, Z.: Effects of maternal attitudes upon improvement in articulation when mothers are trained to assist in speech correction. *J Speech Hear Disord, 29:*126-132, 1964.

Sommers, R., Schaeffer, M., Leiss, R., Gerber, A., Bray, M., Fundrella, D., Olson, J., and Tomkins, E.: The effectiveness of group and individual therapy. *J Speech Hear Res, 9:*219-224, 1966.

Sommers, R., Shilling, S., Paul, C., Copetas, F., Bowser, D., and McClintock, C.: Training parents of children with functional misarticulation. *J Speech Hear Res, 2:*258-265, 1959.

Tufts, L. and Holliday, A.: Effectiveness of trained parents as speech therapists. *J Speech Hear Disord, 24:*395-401, 1959.

Van Riper, C.: *Speech Correction: Principles and Methods.* Englewood Cliffs, P-H, 1972.

Van Riper, C. and Irwin, J.: *Voice and Articulation.* Englewood Cliffs, P-H, 1958.
Weber, J.: Patterning of deviant articulation behavior. *J Speech Hear Disord,* *35:*135-141, 1970.
West, R., Ansberry, M., and Carr, A.: *The Rehabilitation of Speech.* New York, Har-Row, 1937.
Weston, A. and Irwin, J.: Use of paired-stimuli in modification of articulation. *J Percept Motor Skills, 32:*947-957, 1971.
Winitz, H.: *From Syllable to Conversation.* Baltimore, Univ Park, 1975.

CHAPTER 7

Neurogenic Articulation Disorders

I N LIGHT OF THE UNIQUE characteristics of neurogenic articulation defects and the manifest requirements for differential
approaches to therapy, some special attention seems warranted.
However, since there are a number of excellent publications
available on the subject, the material presented here will not be
highly detailed nor totally comprehensive. The discussion is
designed only to introduce the reader to the subject matter and
to outline some clinical approaches to the disorders. For more
indepth coverage the reader is encouraged to consult Darley,
Aronson, and Brown's definitive text, *Motor Speech Disorders*
(Saunders, 1975), and an excellent new edited text by Johns,
Clinical Management of Neurogenic Communicative Disorders (Little,
Brown 1978).

APRAXIA OF SPEECH

The term *apraxia*, in general, refers to a disturbance of purposive motor planning that results from a cortical level lesion
affecting the motor memory center for particular movements. It
is generally believed that the cortex contains, in different locations, memory centers that store the motor plans or "programs"
needed to accomplish specific motor tasks, typically learned
during childhood. Damage to one of these centers may result in a
particular type of apraxia, e.g. limb apraxia, oral apraxia, or
apraxia of speech. The resulting motor disturbance may differ
depending upon severity but cannot be accounted for in terms of
muscular paralysis, incoordination, or altered muscle tone.
Apraxic disorders are typically characterized by an apparent
disparity between relatively normal or on-target movements that
occur automatically, reflexively, or without planning and the
disturbed, off-target movements that accompany purposive,

volitional attempts at particular motor tasks. The relatively normal automatic movements attest to the integrity of the patient's neuromotor system below the level of conscious motor planning. While apraxic conditions may coexist with disorders of muscular paresis, the resultant disturbance in motor ability is typically more involved than would be expected from the paresis alone and, again, the automatic-volitional disparity is diagnostically indicative of the presence of the disorder.

Apraxia of speech (AOS) is a neurogenic articulation disorder that may be differentially diagnosed from dysarthria or aphasia (Johns and Darley, 1970). The disorder has been referenced with a number of labels throughout history. The present name has been in popular use for approximately the last ten years. The consensus is that it is a disorder of purposive speech programming that results from a lesion to the third frontal convolution of the left hemisphere of the brain (Broca's Area). Although AOS may occur concomitantly with dysarthria and aphasia, it may also be found in pure form.

Furthermore, it may coexist with an *oral apraxia,* a condition in which a patient will have difficulty in carrying out purposive movements of the oral articulators of a nonspeech nature. Patients with oral apraxia may experience difficulty when attempting to protrude their tongue on command and when attempting such tasks as pretending to blow out a match. At the same time, the oral apraxic may be observed to perform these acts in a completely normal manner and without difficulty when done automatically without preplanning, i.e. when licking his lips or blowing out a real match. Despite a reasonably high co-occurrence rate, AOS is obviously a different disorder, involving difficulty in articulatory programming for speech.

A good deal of clinical research concerned with the characteristics of AOS has been completed in the past ten years (Johns and Darley, 1970; Aten, Johns, and Darley, 1971; Deal and Darley, 1972; LaPointe and Johns, 1975; Trost and Canter, 1974; Yoss and Darley, 1974; Rosenbek, Wertz and Darley, 1973; Wertz, Rosenbek, and Collins, 1976; and others). Collectively, these clinician-investigators provide us with a rather consistent picture of the symptom complex typifying the patient with AOS. Symptoms or characteristics that have been reported by more than one investigator include the following:

1. Articulation errors are highly inconsistent and un-predictable in occurrence.
2. Articulation errors occur more frequently with affri-cates, fricatives, and consonant clusters.
3. Although all types of errors may be present, sub-stitution errors are the most prevalent.
4. Single feature errors involving a single place dimen-sion are the most common although errors are not always of the simplification type, e.g. intrusion and unrelated substitution errors frequently occur.
5. Articulation is characterized by effortful, off-target groping behavior with false starts, stops, and repeti-tions.
6. Articulation errors occur more frequently on the initial phoneme in words.
7. Articulation errors increase in frequency of occur-rence with increased word length.
8. Articulation errors are frequently anticipatory or metathetic in nature while others are perseverative.
9. Patients are generally aware of and in some cases may anticipate their errors but have difficulty correcting them.
10. Greater articulatory difficulty is experienced during reading and, in some cases, in imitative activity than in spontaneous speech.
11. Some patients are able to improve articulatory accu-racy if given an opportunity to produce more than one response per stimulation.
12. Diadochokinetic syllable rate may be within normal limits for monosyllable repetitions but great difficulty may be observed with attempts at polysyllabic repeti-tions.
13. Prosodic disturbances such as inappropriate juncture, equal and even stress, unusual intonation contours, and abnormal phoneme durations may be observed.

14. Articulation errors occur more frequently on initial phonemes and in words with less frequency of occurrence in the language.
15. Articulation errors occur more frequently on phonemes with posterior place of articulation features than on phonemes with anterior placements.
16. Voiceless for voiced substitution errors are more common than the reverse.
17. Articulatory accuracy may be better in some patients when a combined auditory and visual stimulation is employed.
18. Articulatory accuracy is better for meaningful than nonmeaningful productions.
19. Articulatory accuracy decreases as the distance between successive points or placements of the articulators increases, e.g. more difficulty may be expected in a context involving a movement from a labial to linguapalatal placement than from a linguaalveolar to a linguapalatal posturing.
20. Articulatory accuracy is significantly better in automatic-reactive productions than in purposive-volitional speech.

While all of the above characteristics have been reported to occur in AOS, not all patients will evidence all symptoms. Variability might reasonably be expected depending upon such factors as severity and the coexistence of other disorders, such as aphasia, dysarthria, or oral apraxia. Each patient must be individually evaluated in order to determine the exact phonetic nature of the disorder and the degree to which various stimulus conditions, as listed above, affect articulatory accuracy.

Each clinician may design his own AOS test battery based on activities that will reveal the degree to which the above phonetic and nonphonetic variables influence a specific patient's articulation. However, Wertz (1978) has proposed a test battery that may be of help to the novice clinician. Proposed activities include having the patient do the following: (1) produce isolated vowels; (2) repeat monosyllables and monosyllable combinations; (3) repeat multisyllable words and words of increasing length, such as "please-pleasing-pleasingly"; (4) produce words containing the same initial and final phoneme, such as coke, dad, gag, etc.; (5) repeat sentences, possibly varying in length and phonetic complexity; (6) describe pictures and repeat error sentences made during the spontaneous description; and (7) count from one to twenty and name the days of the week, first forward and then backwards.

Such activities may reveal the presence of the disorder, its phonetic nature, and the degree to which it is affected by the "typical" influences. For example, we might expect the patient to have greater difficulty in producing the monosyllable combinations than the isolated vowels or single monosyllable repetitions. We would expect increasing articulatory difficulty with increasing word length, relative to number three above, and more errors on the initial phoneme than on the final in task number four above. The picture description task provides a spontaneous speech sample and having the patient repeat sentences containing errors should provide an index of the degree to which spontaneous and imitative response modes differ. Automatic activities, such as counting forward and naming the days of the week, should result in better articulation than the less automatic tasks of producing these sequences backward. To this basic test battery we might wish to add a reading task in order to compare articulatory accuracy during reading, spontaneous speech, and under imitative conditions. Further, we may wish to include a word or syllable repetition task designed specifically for the purpose of assessing the degree to which various phonetic environments influence articulatory accuracy. McDonald's Deep Test may be used to partially determine this.

AOS is fundamentally a phonetic level disorder and, as such, the focus of therapy will naturally be on production and production drills. However, the approach taken and the materials used should be determined by the information obtained during assessment. The first few sessions should probably have somewhat of a diagnostic focus since it is usually not possible to obtain all of the necessary information in the initial assessment session. Rosenbek (1978) outlines seven basic factors that need to be considered in planning therapy for a patient with AOS. These include the stimuli to be used, the stimulus and response modes to be employed, the temporal relationships between stimulus presentation and the patient's response, the selection of facilitators and reinforcements, and the method to be employed.

Each of these require a decision by the clinician in designing therapy. The choices should be based upon the information obtained during assessment. As a general rule of thumb, therapy should progress from easier to more difficult levels, with modifications in design as success is achieved. However, increasing the complexity of the stimulus material, difficulty of the response mode, etc., should only be done when there is a good expectation for success.

Depending upon the severity of the disorder and the specific abilities of the patient, the selection of the initial stimulus material may vary anywhere from nonspeech articulatory posturing to complex speech units having differential stress requirements. Work on isolated phonemes might progress from vowels to plosives, nasals, liquids, fricatives and, finally, to affricates and consonant clusters. Within each class, the progression might be from phonemes with anterior place of articulation to those with more posterior locations. Also, voiceless phonemes may be easier than their voiced cognates. Therapy at the word level should begin with short, common VC or CVC words with the target phoneme in the final position. As accuracy improves, CVC words with the target phoneme in the initial position should be introduced. Gradually, the phonetic requirements in the words may be increased and polysyllabic words may be introduced. Finally, the clinician may introduce phrases and sentences varying in phonetic complexity.

In designing therapy the clinician must also decide on the nature or mode of presentation. He may present stimuli through the visual, auditory, or tactile modalities. Whether it is better to use a single modality or a combination approach is somewhat unclear and probably varies with each patient. The clinician must, therefore, determine which stimulus mode or combination is best for each patient. While there does not appear to be a consensus on the matter, the author's own opinion is that all three should probably be used with slightly different emphasis at different stages of therapy. For example, during the early stages of therapy with patients having at least a moderate degree of impairment, emphasizing visual and tactile stimulations through "mirror work" and sensorimotor training has proven effective. During the later stages of therapy and with less involved patients, auditory and visual stimulations seem to be more appropriate.

In all but the most severe cases, the primary response mode should be oral-verbal. However, in some patients the use of a concomitant written or gestural response may facilitate the oral response in certain stages of therapy. The simultaneous or prepatory use of writing and gesturing should be given a clinical trial with each patient to determine potential benefit. Activities should be structured in order to allow for a systematic progression from more automatic responses to ones requiring more planning or purposiveness. Thus, an initial imitative response paradigm should be employed with a gradual fading of the clinician's oral-verbal model. Of course the ultimate objective is articulatory accuracy in spontaneous connected speech. Johns and Darley (1970) suggest that patients be allowed three consecutive responses per stimulation. While this suggestion has been debated, it would appear to be a clinically sound approach, providing the patient with an opportunity for trial and error rehearsal and self-correction.

Whether or not the clinician should enforce a time interval between stimulation and response has not been resolved through hard research data. It is possible that a short delay of one to three seconds might provide the patient with an opportunity to rehearse the speech stimuli subvocally and, thus, increase articulatory accuracy. Again, this might be tested during the early stages of therapy in order to determine potential usefulness with a given patient.

Rosenbek (1978) suggests that a number of suprasegmental, prosodic elements of speech may function as facilitators and increase the likelihood of correct responses. These include novel variations in loudness, pitch, articulation, and pause time and differential stress. In presenting stimuli, clinicians may wish to initially utilize one or more of these emphasizing or highlighting techniques in eliciting responses. However, as success is achieved, these should be faded in favor of a more natural speech prosody. An approach based almost solely on the use of prosody to rebuild expressive speech skills is *melodic intonation therapy*. The interested reader is referred to a 1974 article by Sparks, Helm, and Albert.

The specific therapy method selected is at the discretion of the individual clinician. Since AOS is a phonetically based articulation disorder, any of the techniques or approaches discussed in Chapter 6 that are appropriate to such disorders may be used with an expectation of success, given that the above considerations are included in the design. More than one approach may be used at different stages of therapy. For example, phonetic placement, progressive approximation, the key word method, sensorimotor techniques, etc., may all be appropriately applied with different patients or during different stages of treatment. It is, of course, necessary to modify suggested procedures inherent in some of these approaches in order to arrange the stimuli and design the therapy program in accord with the phonetic and nonphonetic factors that influence production accuracy. Therapy for AOS may be a rewarding experience for both the client and clinician. When the general guidelines discussed here are followed and adapted to the individual patient's needs, progress can normally be expected. The author's clinical experience suggests that, in all but the most severe cases, when therapy is initiated early after onset of the disorder the prognosis for significant gains with therapy is good.

DEVELOPMENTAL AOS

The preceding discussion on apraxia of speech was concerned primarily with a disorder occurring generally in adulthood due to an acquired lesion. Acquired AOS generally results from easily discernable etiologies, such as stroke, head injury, tumor, infectious diseases, or neurotoxicity. However, it is becoming increasingly obvious that many children with moderate and severe articulation disorders evidence characteristics that warrant a differential diagnosis of *developmental apraxia of speech*. Developmental AOS is not as easily diagnosed as acquired AOS in adults. This is probably due to the fact that (1) the phonological systems in such children have not matured, resulting in both phonetic and phonemic errors and (2) the neuropathology is less clear and typically ill-defined. Nonetheless, the author is convinced that the disorder is a very real entity and that such children require special treatment programs.

Yoss and Darley (1974) examined thirty school-aged children with moderate and severe articulation defects. Their examination battery included a number of speech and nonspeech tasks. Of the thirty children examined, sixteen were identified as having characteristics that separated them from the others and, according to the authors, warranted the label of developmental AOS. Many of the reported characteristics are similar to those typically found in adults with acquired AOS, such as (1) reduced diadochokinetic ability with special difficulty producing three syllable combinations (often resulting in metathetic syllable errors), (2) greater difficulty with polysyllabic words, with errors of omission, addition-intrusion and sound and syllable revision, (3) an occasional prosodic disturbance characterized by slower speech rate, equalized stress, and restricted pitch, and (4) difficulty with volitional oral movements, especially those involving the tongue and lips.

However, Yoss and Darley report that unlike acquired AOS in adults, children with developmental AOS differ in four ways: (1) they usually have an accompanying oral apraxia; (2) they do not evidence the audible groping and effortful trial and error behavior typical of acquired AOS; (3) they do not appear to be aware of their errors unless they are older or have received extensive speech therapy; and (4) they have a higher incidence of multiple feature errors and distortion errors in spontaneous speech. In addition to the above, Yoss and Darley report that these children have a high incidence of neurological soft signs, such as disturbed fine motor coordination, awkward gait, and alternate motion rates of the extremities and tongue. They suggest that specific learning disabilities may or may not accompany developmental AOS. They also report a high incidence of poor auditory perception, especially auditory sequencing, but suggest that these findings are also common in children with non-AOS articulatory defects.

Rosenbek and Wertz (1972) reviewed fifty cases of developmental AOS and suggest the following symptoms as diagnostically indicative: (1) the presence of vowel errors; (2) the presence of oral apraxia; (3) an increase in errors with longer productions; and (4) groping postures of the speech muscles. Others, like Haynes, Johns, and May (1978), suggest a high occurrence of orosensory perceptual deficits in developmental AOS. These authors urge clinicians to include tests of orosensory perception in their test batteries for developmental AOS.

Haynes (1978) provides an excellent summary of the current knowledge of developmental AOS and the reader is encouraged to consult her contribution for a more detailed picture than is presented here. She suggests that the test battery should include tools for the assessment of the following: (1) language ability, in light of the high incidence of delayed speech and language development in such children and the possible coexistence of congenital aphasia; (2) articulatory proficiency and the phonetic influences previously discussed; (3) oral diadochokineses; (4) volitional movements of the oral musculature; and (5) orosensory perception.

As with the acquired disorder in adults, therapy for developmental AOS must be tailored to the individual child and the manifest symptoms. Many of the considerations and techniques discussed in the preceding section may be directly applicable to children with developmental AOS. Haynes suggests a number of activities that may be quite useful with selected patients: (1) concentrated, nonspeech tongue and lip placement and movement drills for the purpose of improving volitional movement capability; (2) imitation of sustained vowels and consonants, gradually moving to simple syllable shapes; (3) using a slow speech articulation rate in order to increase the awareness of sensorimotor patterns involved in producing speech movement sequences and to heighten self-monitoring ability; (4) establishing a key word core vocabulary; (5) using stereotyped carrier phrases with different word completions, e.g. "I want a . . . ," in order to establish articulatory sequencing at the sentence level; (6) using rhythm, intonation, and differential stress in order to facilitate motor sequencing; and (7) using a series of tactile stimulation activities in order to heighten orosensory perceptual awareness. Haynes also suggests that frequent (daily) and intensive therapy drill sessions are best and that referral for possible physical therapy, audiological and psychological services may be warranted for many of these children.

It is felt that many children with moderate and severe articulation disorders, at least a significant minority of those comprising speech pathologists' caseloads, have characteristics indicative of developmental apraxia of speech. These children are generally quite resistant to the traditional articulation therapy approaches often taken by unaware clinicians. It is important for speech pathologists to be aware of the AOS syndrome in children so that they may be appropriately identified and treated.

DYSARTHRIA

While this book would be incomplete without some discussion of the dysarthrias, the author is somewhat reticent to address the subject because the breadth of the topic goes far beyond the limitations imposed on it by a small section of one chapter. Further, dysarthria is a multifaceted disorder that may involve all aspects of speech, not just articulation. Nonetheless, an attempt will be made to introduce the reader to the subject and to discuss, in general, some treatment considerations. It is assumed that the student will receive individual coursework on the subject and that the references cited will be reviewed for in-depth coverage.

First, it is important to say that *dysarthria* is the generic term that refers to any isolated or combined disturbance of respiration, phonation, resonance, or articulation that results from nervous system damage. The speech disturbance(s) is directly attributable to defective neuromotor strength, coordination, or muscle tone. Thus, we may use the term when referring to the defective speech of a cerebral palsied child or an adult with an acquired neuropathology.

The particular characteristics of dysarthria and the specific speech processes affected will depend upon the location and extent of the damage to the nervous system. A number of classification systems have been designed. The one that has received the widest acceptance in speech pathology was proposed by Darley, Aronson and Brown (1969).

These authors suggest that there are at least six major types of dysarthria that may be differentially identified by the practicing speech pathologist: (1) *flaccid dysarthria,* characterized by a breathy voice quality, hypernasality, and consonant imprecision;

(2) *spastic dysarthria,* typically characterized by a strained, harsh voice quality, variable hypernasality, and imprecise articulation; (3) *ataxic dysarthria,* characterized by disturbed prosody, imprecise consonant articulations and irregular articulatory breakdowns; (4) *hypokinetic dysarthria,* as in Parkinson's disease, characterized by short "rushes of speech," restricted pitch and loudness, imprecise consonants, and inappropriate silences; (5) *hyperkinetic dysarthria,* characterized by involuntary articulatory or phonatory gestures or movements, distorted vowels, imprecise consonant articulations, prolonged intervals of silence, harsh or strained voice quality, variability in rate, irregular articulatory breakdown, and restricted pitch and loudness usage; and (6) *mixed dysarthria,* characterized by two or more of the above symptom clusters.

Of course, the above symptoms may vary for a given patient depending upon the severity of the dysarthria and the extent of involvement of the four primary speech processes. For example, in the case of a severe flaccid paralysis involving all of the cranial nerves, the patient may not be able to phonate at all due to complete bilateral vocal fold paralysis, may evidence shallow, weak respiration, and may not be able to hold his head erect because of a weak neck musculature. He may also have difficulty swallowing (dysphagia), manifest drooling, and may be totally unable to move the articulators (tongue, lips, soft palate) in a manner requisite for even minimal speech production. On the other hand, a patient with a mild flaccid paresis restricted in terms of cranial nerve involvement, may manifest only slight articulatory difficulty with the motorically more difficult consonant phonemes or may evidence only an isolated, slight breathy quality. Thus, the symptoms vary widely even within a given classification or type of dysarthria.

It is important for the speech pathologist to complete a thorough examination of each patient and to delineate the extent and type of neuromotor involvement affecting the basic processes of speech. Only in this way may therapy be individualized. A complete oral peripheral examination (see Chapter 5) and a good understanding of physiological phonetics are the best tools for clinical assessment. The reader should consult the works of Darley, Aronson, and Brown (1975) and Johns (1978) for detailed discussions of diagnostic methods.

Speech therapy is designed primarily to help the dysarthric patient compensate for the underlying neuromotor disturbance. That is, the goal of therapy should be to assist the patient in maximizing speech intelligibility within the limitations of his neuromotor capabilities. While some nonspeech oral exercises may help the patient to gain an awareness of the articulators and basic movement patterns, oral gymnastics solely for the purpose of strengthening the musculature is probably a waste of time. The author is not of the opinion that "physical therapy of the mouth" is an effective approach.

Therapy activities that may be beneficial are described below under each of the three major headings.

1. *Articulation Therapy* should be initiated with a program of discrimination training in order to make the patient aware of his articulation difficulty. The focus should be on developing both an auditory and, where feasible, orosensory awareness of articulation. This should be accompanied by clinician explanations of the problem and cause of the difficulty. Activities designed to slow rate of speech to an optimum level and increase the accuracy of individual phoneme articulations should be employed. Exaggerating consonant and, where needed, vowel articulations may help develop an awareness of correct phonetic posturing for the more difficult phonemes. A syllable by syllable attack may help slow rate of speech and improve articulatory precision. Individual phonemes should be worked on in a variety of syllable contexts with exaggerated and prolonged movements to emphasize the sensorimotor aspects of correct articulation. With success, work should focus on polysyllabic words with emphasis on the medial and final syllables. Finally, work at the connected speech level should emphasize self-monitoring relative to appropriate rate, articulatory accuracy, and speech intelligibility.

2. *Phonation and Respiration.* These two basic motor processes should be worked on together. Therapy, where needed, should be designed to establish an optimum pitch and loudness level and to improve voice quality. Some attention may be paid to increasing pitch and loudness range or variability. Standard voice therapy techniques may be applied. The use of pitch and loudness meters and other feedback devices may be most appropriate. In case of laryngeal hypertonicity, work on developing an easier initiation of phonation and establishing a pattern of some aspiration prior to phonation may be helpful. In the case of flaccidity and laryngeal hypotonicity, techniques designed to encourage increased vocal fold tension, such as having the patient attempt hard glottal attacks and pushing exercises, may be beneficial. In order to compensate for an inadequate breath support, the patient may be encouraged to speak at higher lung volumes and to shorten individual productions. Some work on phrasing may be needed. For example, productions may be best when the patient produces only three or four words, or less, per exhalation. Experimentation to determine optimal phrasing should be conducted. Disturbed respiration should be viewed in terms of the effect on phonation.

3. *Resonance Therapy* designed to improve velopharyngeal competency has not been shown to be effective. However, activities such as encouraging the patient to use greater mouth opening and normal tongue posturing may help reduce the extent of hypernasality. Discrimination training may also help the patient to develop an awareness of and, subsequently, reduce the extent of oral-nasal imbalance. Pharyngeal hypertonicity may result in a disturbed voice quality and, in such cases, working with the patient to achieve a more normal or relaxed pharyngeal tonicity may help.

In addition to the above, speech pathologists may wish to consider the possible use of a variety of prostheses that may assist the patient with speech production. In consultation with the physician, physical therapist, occupational therapist, prosthodontist, etc., the speech pathologist may wish to suggest methods, other than speech therapy, to improve the status of the speech mechanism. Such devices as palatal lift prostheses to achieve velopharyngeal closure, teflon injections into the medial surface of a paralyzed vocal fold to allow fold adduction for phonation and the use of a variety of head, neck, and upper body bracing mechanisms to improve posture for speech are examples of potentially helpful prostheses. All options for improvement, including prosthetic, surgical, and therapeutic management, should be considered. The reader may wish to consult the work of Johns and Salyer (1978) for further discussion of possible surgical and prosthetic management techniques. Interprofessional referral and team work should be a routine component of the speech pathologist's work with dysarthric patients.

REFERENCES

Aten, J., Johns, D., and Darley, F.: Auditory perception of sequenced words in apraxia of speech. *J Speech Hear Res, 14:*131, 1971.

Darley, F., Aronson, A., and Brown, J.: Differential diagnostic patterns of dysarthria. *J Speech Hear Res, 12:*246-269, 1969.

Darley, F., Aronson, A., and Brown, J.: *Motor Speech Disorders.* Philadelphia, Saunders, 1975.

Deal, J. and Darley, F.: The influence of linguistic and situational variables on phonemic accuracy in apraxia of speech. *J Speech Hear Res, 15:*639, 1972.

Haynes, S.: Developmental apraxia of speech: symptoms and treatment. In Johns, D. (Ed.): *Clinical Management of Neurogenic Communicative Disorders.* Boston, Little, 1978.

Haynes, S., Johns, D., and May, E.: Assessment and therapeutic management of an adult patient with development apraxia of speech and orosensory perceptual deficits. *Tejas, 3:*6, 1978.

Johns, D.: *Clinical Management of Neurogenic Communicative Disorders.* Boston, Little, 1978.

Johns, D. and Darley, F.: Phonemic variability in apraxia of speech. *J Speech Hear Res, 13:*556, 1970.

Johns, D. and Salyer, K.: Surgical and prosthetic management of neurogenic speech disorders. In Johns, D. (Ed.): *Clinical Management of Neurogenic Communicative Disorders.* Boston, Little, 1978.

LaPointe, L. and Johns, D.: Some phonemic characteristics in apraxia of speech. *J Comm Disord, 8:*259, 1975.

Rosenbek, J.: Treating apraxia of speech. In Johns, D. (Ed.): *Clinical Management of Neurogenic Communicative Disorders.* Boston, Little, 1978.

Rosenbek, J. and Wertz, R.: A review of 50 cases of developmental apraxia of speech. *Lang Speech Hear Serv Schools, 3:*23, 1972.

Rosenbek, J., Wertz, R., and Darley, F.: Oral sensation and perception in apraxia of speech and aphasia. *J Speech Hear Res, 16:*22, 1973.

Sparks, R., Helm, N., and Albert, M.: Aphasia rehabilitation resulting from melodic intonation therapy. *Cortex, 10:*303, 1974.

Trost, J. and Canter, G.: Apraxia of speech in patients with Broca's aphasia: a study of phoneme production accuracy and error patterns. *Brain and Lang, 1:*63, 1974.

Wertz, R.: Neuropathologies of speech and language: an introduction to patient management. In Johns, D. (Ed.): *Clinical Management of Neurogenic Communicative Disorders.* Boston, Little, 1978.

Wertz, R., Rosenbek, J., and Collins, M.: Identification of apraxia of speech from PICA verbal tests. In Wertz, R. and Collins, M. (Eds.): *Clinical Aphasiology: Conference Proceedings, 1972.* Madison, Veterans Administration Hospital, 1976.

Yoss, C. and Darley, F.: Developmental apraxia of speech in children with defective articulation. *J Speech Hear Res, 17:*399, 1974.

CHAPTER 8

Articulation Disorders in the Hearing Impaired

ROBERT D. MOULTON, PH.D.

T HE PRACTICING SPEECH pathologist is probably well aware of the important role that hearing plays in the development of normal speech and language. Indeed, most speech pathologists routinely look for indications in the case history and/or intake interview of factors that would indicate the presence or absence of normal hearing. Furthermore, most speech pathologists consider a hearing screen to be an integral part of the evaluation process. Most of our university training programs stress the causative role that impaired hearing can have on communicative disorders and the speech pathologist and the audiologist are relatively well trained in the need and techniques for the identification of hearing thresholds.

A serious problem exists, however, once a significant hearing loss has been identified. In the opinion of this author, the majority of speech pathologists are not prepared to handle the peculiar speech problems of the hearing impaired. In most of our university programs, academic and clinical training in speech habilitation for the auditorially handicapped are not given the attention that they deserve. The present chapter is written in an attempt to answer such questions as, "what do I do after I have identified a hearing loss? What is the role of the speech pathologist in a habilitation program for the hearing impaired? What are the typical speech problems of the deaf and hard of hearing? How can these typical speech problems be avoided?" While the main thrust of the chapter will be the speech of the deaf, other factors such as language, educational practices, and psycholinguistics will be discussed.

233

POPULATION AND PROGRAMS

One of the first discoveries that the speech pathologist will make when studying the speech of the deaf is that "the deaf" as a population are difficult to delineate. That is, the parameters associated with hearing loss are such that the hearing impaired do not present a homogeneous group. Factors such as type of loss, extent of loss, age at onset of loss, use of amplification, and educational philosophies espoused by parents and school programs all tend to make clear categorization of the hearing handicapped a difficult if not a futile process.

The term *hearing impaired* is usually considered to include a broad range of hearing ability, from the profoundly deaf to the mildly hard of hearing. Between these two extremes lies a broad range of hearing losses and there has traditionally been some disagreement as to how different degrees of hearing loss should be categorized. In 1973, the Conference of Executives of American Schools for the Deaf created the Committee to Redefine Deaf and Hard of Hearing for Educational Purposes and the results of this committee are being used more and more to help classify levels of hearing loss (Frisina, 1974). The Committee defined *deaf* as a hearing loss of at least 70 dB ISO, which precludes the understanding of speech through audition, and *hard of hearing* as a loss of 35 to 69 dB ISO, which makes the understanding of speech through audition difficult, but not impossible.

The Committee also broke levels of hearing loss down into smaller categories for educational placement. Moores (1978) reports these levels to be as follows

1. *Level I, 35 to 54 dB.* Individuals in this category routinely do not require special class/school placement; they routinely do require special speech and hearing assistance.
2. *Level II, 55 to 69 dB.* These individuals occasionally require special class/school placement; they routinely require special speech, hearing, and language assistance.
3. *Level III, 70 to 89 dB.* Those in this category of deafness routinely require special class/school placement; they routinely require special speech, hearing, language, and educational assistance.
4. *Level IV, 90 dB and beyond.* These individuals routinely require special class/school placement; they routinely require special speech, hearing, language, and educational assistance.

It should be noted that Moores is of the opinion that losses greater than 35 dB may affect speech production. While this has also been the experience of the present writer, it should not be concluded that the 35 dB level is the sole determinant for the need for speech habilitation. It should also be mentioned that the above stated levels are considered by some to be too heavily weighted toward the deaf side of the hearing loss continuum. Ross and Giolas (1978), for example, state that an individual should be considered to be hard of hearing if he has a hearing loss between 15 and 100 dB. Ross and Giolas use this exceptionally wide bracket because they believe that with optimal and timely auditory management (amplification, auditory training, etc.) more of the hearing impaired population would make better use of residual hearing and, thus, would behave as hard of hearing rather than deaf.

In this writer's experience, the categories developed by the Committee to Redefine Deaf and Hard of Hearing for Educational Purposes fit closely to the behavior pattern that the speech pathologist can expect. That is, an individual with a loss greater than 70 dB is likely to have the speech and language problems one usually associates with deafness. Whether this would necessarily be the case with optimal auditory management is a topic whose scope is beyond the confines of this chapter.

In addition to degree of hearing loss, the age of onset of the loss is usually considered as an important educational factor. The *prelingually* or *congenitally* deaf individuals are considered to have been born with their hearing loss or to have lost their hearing before speech and language began to develop. Since we now know from research in speech perception and psycholinguistics that even new-born infants react to speech and language patterns differently than they do to other sounds, it may well be that the term *prelingual deafness* in reality refers to deafness at birth and hence the phrase *congenital deafness* is probably more appropriate.

Postlingual deafness refers to a significant hearing loss that occurs after speech and language have already developed through normal auditory channels. The term *adventitiously deaf* has sometimes been used to refer to the *postlingually* deafened. The distinction between the congenitally and postlingually deaf person is an important one. The majority of hearing impaired children in educational programs have hearing losses that are considered to be congenital. The speech pathologist can readily appreciate the fact that speech and language remediation for the congenitally deaf will be an entirely different process from that used with the postlingually deafened.

The categories described thus far have some physical or natural reason for their existence: levels of hearing loss measured in dB and age of onset of loss. A major educational categorization exists, however, that is based on philosophical rather than physical considerations. This grouping concerns the method of communication to be used with the hearing impaired in the home and in educational programming. The speech pathologist who attempts to work with the deaf will soon learn that this philosophical consideration is not taken lightly by parents, teachers, administrators, and the hearing impaired population. In general, the issue involves the use of manual forms of communication and the relative importance that programs give to the development of speech. An overly simplistic view of the different philosophical approaches to educating the deaf would be that one group, the *oralists,* believe that speech and language can best be developed through speechreading and amplification of sound; while the other group, the *total communication* advocates, state that all forms of communication, including signs and fingerspelling, should be used with the hearing impaired. Such a simple view, however, is not sufficient to prepare the speech pathologist for the vehemence, dogmatism, and religious fervor with which proponents of differing philosophies approach educating the deaf.

The speech pathologist may obtain insight into the methodology battle that has permeated deaf education for at least two hundred years by looking at the historical development of the two movements. The split between the oral and manual camps has existed from the very beginnings of deaf education. In fact, the basis for the ideological differences can be traced back to the beginnings of the fields of philosophy, psychology, and education when early leaders in these fields were speculating on the relationship between thought, language, and speech (Boring, 1950). Many of the early questions regarding thought, language, and speech are still providing researchers and educators with topics for investigation, discussion, and at times open confrontation. It is still cogent to ask: "is thought possible without language? Is language possible without speech? Are language and thought the same thing?" Early philosophers concerned themselves with questions such as these and sought to grasp the nature of language, thinking, ideas, speech, words, etc., through introspection and later through semiempirical research (Johnson, 1972). These "black box" investigations, as they have been called, led to the development of several schools of thought. Two of these schools, empiricism and behaviorism, were to have profound implications in education of the deaf.

The *empirical school,* founded by Locke in the 1600s, held that thinking took place in words, which were merely an internal replication of speech. To Locke, language, thought, and the spoken words were simply different manifestations of the same thing (Garnett, 1967). This tenet was also held by Watson, founder of the American Behaviorist Movement. He states that " . . . according to my view, thought processes are really motor habits in the larynx" (Slobin, 1971). There were those, however, who took exception to the empiricists and argued that thought could occur in forms other than speech.

Education of the deaf began in Europe and was later "imported" to the United States. From its very beginnings in Europe, heated controversy existed between the relative roles of speech and sign language in the development of language and thinking. Samuel Heinicke (1729-1748), an early proponent of the oral method in Germany, was influenced by the empirical philosophy and held that thinking was a form of inner speech (Garnett, 1967). Heinicke believed that, since thinking was composed of speech patterns, deaf children must learn speech in order to think. He rejected any form of manual communication and held that only through spoken language patterns was abstract reasoning possible.

The early proponents of the manual system countered these claims by stating that manual signs took the place of words in the thinking process. The Abbé Charles Michel de l'Epeé, who founded the first school for the deaf using the language of signs in 1775, claimed that signs, not words, were the "mother tongue" of the deaf and were used in the thinking and language process (Bender, 1960). De l'Epeé and Heinicke were contemporaries and both appear to have loved a good fight as long as a considerable distance separated the protagonists. They began a series of heated written debates over the relative merits of speech and signs and the published versions of their exchanges only served to increase the polarity between the oral and manual camps. It was from this atmosphere of division that deaf education was exported to the United States.

Since arriving in the United States, the two forms have undergone some metamorphosis, but the same basis for disagreement remains. Currently, programs for the deaf follow educational philosophies that usually fall into one of the following classifications:

1. *Oral.* In this method, children are taught speech and language through speechreading and sound amplification. Sign language and fingerspelling are not allowed since the proponents of the method believe that manual forms of communication preclude speech, speechreading, and audition.
2. *Total Communication.* This philosophy stresses a multitude of communication options for the child. Sign language, gesture, fingerspelling, auditory training, speechreading, speech, mime, reading, writing, etc., are used in the home and school by the child, parent, and educator. Family members and teachers are expected to be proficient in manual communication modes and these modes are expected to be used simultaneously with audible speech that should be amplified via hearing aids or auditory training units.
3. *Rochester Method.* This method is not used much in the United States at present but a method similar to it is used in the Soviet Union. The method is perhaps best described as a combination of oralism and fingerspelling. Parents and educators are expected to speak in complete sentences while fingerspelling every word. This sounds difficult but the proficient fingerspeller can communicate with the manual al-

phabet at about the same rate that a first class secretary can type (80 to 100 words per minute). The reasoning behind the method is that if every word is finger-spelled, the child will receive an intact language model. Also, it is felt that the transition from the manual alphabet letters to phones for speech is not a difficult one.

4. *Cued Speech*. This system attracted a few followers in the late sixties and early seventies but has few disciples now. Developed by Doctor Orin Cornett, the cued speech method was seen as a compromise between oral and manual methods. It consists of a phonetic alphabet and a manual alphabet code system that is incomplete without lipreading. The hearing impaired receiver of a cued message would have to rely on both lipreading and the manual code to understand the message.

5. *Auditory-Only or Oral/Aural Method*. This system would appear at this moment to be gaining some impetus, especially in oral programs that are taking a renewed interest in auditory training. This method stresses early identification and amplification and seeks to lessen the dependence on visual means of communication such as sign language *and* speechreading. The idea is that by removing visual input the hearing impaired child will more readily come to rely on residual hearing.

As with most categorizations, there is often not a clear dichotomy between programs and at times a difference exists between the "official" philosophy of an educational program and what is practiced. The writer has seen many "oral or oral/aural" programs where manual forms of communication were used by the children, some of the teachers, most of the dormitory staff, and many of the parents. While visiting a program that was proported to be using the Rochester Method, the writer was chagrined to see that while the school administration relied on fingerspelling, the faculty and students used what may best be described as total communication.

Because of this lack of a clear distinction between philosophies in many programs, it is difficult to acquire an accurate picture of how the hearing impaired are educated in the United States. Probably the best estimate has been reported by Jorday, Gustason, and Rosen in 1976. These researchers surveyed 7,181 classes for the hearing handicapped and indicate that total communication is the most frequently reported educational philosophy (64%). The oral philosophy is espoused by 33 percent of the respondents and the Rochester and Cued Speech Programs accounted for about 3 percent. In addition, Jordan et al., report that a shift toward greater numbers of total communication classes is occurring.

The point of all of this is that while all of the educational philosophies have intelligible and pleasant speech as a goal, the methods by which they attempt to reach this goal may differ. Depending on the work setting, the speech pathologist may find differing opinions concerning the merits of sign language, auditory training, early amplification, speechreading, fingerspelling, etc. These differing opinions are *not* to be taken lightly. The speech pathologist practicing his profession in a total communication setting should be aware that fluent manual communication skills are a must for all who work with the children within that system. Sadly, the majority of our professional training programs in speech pathology do not include manual communication skills and experience in their training package. On the other hand, the speech pathologist employed in an oral or oral/aural school should realize that the school's and parents' policy against sign language and fingerspelling is not usually a negotiable item open for discussion. Also, the speech pathologist contemplating employment in an oral or oral/aural setting should be aware that the typical university training program has probably not prepared him for the great and complex type and amount of auditory training that he will be expected to provide for the children.

In addition to educational philosophy, differences exist between programs relative to educational location. That is, some classes for the hearing impaired are located in relatively large *residential schools* while others may be found in *day schools* or within regular public schools where the hearing handicapped are more or less *mainstreamed*. Rawlings and Trybus (1978) report the program types to be as follows:

TABLE VIII

PERSONNEL, FACILITIES AND SERVICES AVAILABLE IN SCHOOLS AND CLASSES FOR HEARING IMPAIRED CHILDREN IN THE UNITED STATES

Program Type	Number of Programs	Total Enrollment	% of Total Enrollment	Median Enrollment
Residential Schools for the Deaf	69	19,521	32%	256
Residential Schools for the Multiply Handicapped	41	2,435	4%	37
Day Schools for the deaf	76	7,513	12%	60
Day Schools for the Multiply Handicapped	25	2,349	4%	35
School Districts Offering Full-Time Classes Only	129	4,365	7%	17
School Districts Offering Part Time Classes and Services	436	24,138	40%	25
Total All Programs	776	60,231	100%	

SOURCE: Brenda W. Rawlings and Raymond J. Trybus, Personnel, Facilities and Services Available in Schools and classes for Hearing Impaired Children in the United States, *American Annals for the Deaf, 123:*99-114, 1978.

This means that the speech pathologist who works with the hearing handicapped may be placed in work settings that could differ in program type or location as well as in philosophy. When considering program type, the speech pathologist needs to be aware of several factors. Note in Table VIII that the median enrollment for the residential schools is at least five or six times greater than day school or regular public school mainstream programs. This means that the residential schools usually have the advantages of larger student numbers from which to make homogeneous groupings, supervisory staff experienced in deaf education, and often more financial resources (Brill, Merrill, and Frisina, 1973). On the other hand, there is much to be said for day schools and other forms of local programming that allow children to remain at home and to have a more "normal" environment with hearing peers to provide models and motivation for speech and language.

Rawlings and Trybus (1978) report that about 69,000 hearing

impaired individuals are receiving services in special educational classrooms in the United States in nearly 800 different programs. They further note that 54 percent of these programs have at least one full-time speech pathologist and 29 percent of the programs have at least one part-time speech pathologist. This means that a great majority of the educational settings for the hearing impaired have the services of a speech pathologist. At present, however, no hard data is available as to the type, amount, or efficacy of these services. We are also unable to specify the levels and types of certification and training of the speech pathologists providing the services.

SPEECH DEVELOPMENT

The above discussion should make it clear that the diversity of the variables associated with the hearing impaired population make it very difficult to make any definitive statements regarding speech development, speech problems, or speech correction of the hearing handicapped. Because of this, this writer has elected to address himself to one end of the hearing-nonhearing spectrum: the deaf or severely hard of hearing. The reader is asked to keep in mind that in most cases the individuals with greater levels of hearing loss will have relatively more speech problems. Also, the course of speech development will usually deviate more from the norm in those children with greater losses of hearing. The speech pathologist can assume that the following discussion is specific to the deaf population and adjustments in expectations and training modes will have to be made for those with better hearing ability.

In 1978, Donald Moores produced a definitive treatise on deafness. The book, *Educating the Deaf* (Houghton Mifflin Company, 1978), will, in the opinion of this writer, eventually be considered a classic. In discussing speech for the deaf, Moores decries the fact that "educators of the deaf, as a group, make no distinction between speech development and speech remediation." In practice, this is probably true, but the literature on speech for the deaf does contain considerable discussion on the topic. In most cases, however, research on speech development for the hearing impaired is equivocal and "scholarly" discussions and opinions on the subject usually do not correlate well with contemporary knowledge in speech science, linguistics, and psycholinguistics.

In writing about speech for the hearing impaired, many authors do not make a clear distinction between *speech development* and *language development*. This is most evident in the book by Mildred Groht, *Natural Language for Deaf Children* (Alexander Graham Bell, 1958). This book has become a classic and the suggestions for speech and language development it contains have come to be known as the *Natural Method*. In short, the tenets of the Natural Method suggest that both speech and language are the result of a need to communicate. Groht contends that if you provide the deaf child with enough varied and exciting experiences, the child will have such a need to communicate that speech and language will be the "natural" result. It is the role of the teacher, parent, speech pathologist, etc., according to the Natural Method, to provide the child with experience situations and then to give the child the necessary speech and language to express the concepts derived from the situation. In one form or another, nearly all of the current methods or philosophies for teaching the hearing impaired incorporate the Natural Method. That is, using experiences and concepts as a base from which to build speech and the language is an important part of most educational programs. A notable exception to this is the Association Method, which will be discussed later.

The speech pathologist may find that many of the parents of severely hearing impaired children have received information and/or training in speech development philosophy and techniques through the John Tracy Correspondence Course or Clinic. The John Tracy program is designed to help parents of deaf children through the child's first five years of life. The correspondence course and clinic were founded by Mrs. Spencer Tracy because of her concern for deaf children and their parents. Mrs. Tracy's concern was in part fostered by her experiences with her deaf son, John, for whom the program is named. Parents of hearing impaired children can receive free information and advice through the mail or they may travel to California and stay at the clinic for a training program. The philosophy of the program is decidedly oral and the information presented closely follows the Natural Method. The program has been especially helpful to parents living in areas remote from speech/hearing/deaf education centers. This writer knows of no equivalent program for parents who wish to begin total communication at an early age.

While there is considerable agreement for the idea that experiences and concepts should form the basis for speech and language development, there is very little agreement on how speech and language interact. That is, once the experience and concept phase has been completed, considerable conflict exists concerning how the language for the concept should be presented to the child and how speech should be encouraged. The oralists contend that language can be presented via speechreading and/or audition and that speech develops from a combination of imitation of the visual and amplified auditory model. In this writer's experience, most oral programs rely on various combinations of tactual, visual, auditory, and kinesthetic cues to present the speech models for the expression of the language experience. Total communication advocates, on the other hand, contend that speechreading and audition are insufficient channels of communication for most hearing impaired children and that more efficient means are needed to transmit the language model for the experiences and concepts. Total communication programs contend that gestures, sign language, fingerspelling, pantomime, etc., can be added to speechreading and audition to convey the language and that once a language system has been established, the language system itself can be used to initiate the speech development process.

Contemporary writers have been more specific than Groht concerning how speech is developed in the hearing impaired child. Most notable have been the recent works of Daniel Ling. Doctor Ling and his wife, Agnes, have been prolific writers on speech for the hearing impaired and on aural habilitation. They spend considerable time presenting workshops; "Doing the Ling Thing" in speech and auditory training has had a tremendous impact on deaf education during the past few years. In his book, *Speech and the Hearing Impaired Child* (Alexander Graham Bell, 1976), Ling outlines in detail what he considers to be the stages of speech development in the hearing impaired:

Essentially, then, there appear to be five broad, mainly sequential stages through which children must, and normally do, pass as they develop speech production skills. The patterns produced in each of the five stages may be described as: (1) undifferentiated vocalization; (2) non-segmental voice patterns varied in duration, intensity, and pitch; (3) a range of distinctly different vowel sounds; (4) simple consonants releasing, modifying, or arresting syllables; and (5) consonant blends.

Note that Ling is concerned here with speech production rather than the language component of communication. It is apparent that he has taken the phonetic aspects of speech, broken them down into subtasks, and developed a hierarchical order. Ling contends that each step of his hierarchy of development is a necessary one and that the teacher, parent, or speech pathologist should not proceed to a higher stage until each successive stage has been mastered. A unique aspect of Ling's philosophy of speech development of the deaf is his advocacy of phonetic drill. Most writers on this subject contend that speech development activities should be phonologic in character and should stress useful phrases and sentences (Ewing and Ewing, 1964; Calvert and Silverman, 1975; Groht, 1958; Di Carlo, 1964). In reviewing the writings of Ling, particularly the five stages described above, one might well ask, as did Moores, if what is discussed might more properly be described as speech remediation rather than speech development.

Several writers on speech development for the deaf have attempted to use normal speech acquisition milestones as a matrix. It is customary for such writers to make reference to the early speculation by speech and hearing authors that speech development flows from reflexive vocalization to babbling, lalling, echolalia, and finally results in true speech. These developmental milestones are used, along with age brackets stated in months, as the framework for describing goals and related activities for speech development in deaf children (Sitnick, Rushmer, and Arpan, 1978; Fry, 1978; and Calvert and Silverman, 1975). Many of the larger residential schools for the deaf and some state educational agencies have adopted a speech development curriculum and, in this writer's experience, most of these curricula follow the "milestone match" formula. Usually, these guidelines suggest that a deaf child, with optimal assistance from the family, proper amplification, normal intelligence, etc., should coo or lall between zero and three months, babble at about six months, begin imitation and echolalic behavior between seven and nine months, and produce single words between ten and twelve months.

Many curricula and authors go one step further and specify a *phoneme development hierarchy*. With a phoneme development hierarchy, a list of phonemes to "teach" is presented with a suggested sequential order. As might be expected, the specific order of phoneme acquisition is not universally agreed upon. Some hierarchies have been based on the classic studies of Wellman et al. (1931), Poole (1934), or Templin (1952 and 1957) that attempt to specify the developmental order of phoneme acquisition by hearing children. Calvert, Davis, and Silverman (1975) present a phoneme development order based on estimated ease of production. Other hierarchies, such as those developed by Yale (1938) and McGinnis (1963), appear to be based solely on the experience or "logic" of the author. The very existence of a phoneme developmental order seems to encourage teachers and parents to teach phonemes in isolation and to approach speech development in the hearing impaired from an overly simplistic motoric or phonetic attitude.

The *Yale* or *Northampton* system has remained a popular framework for speech development and is used in many schools for the deaf as a developmental hierarchy for phonemes. Indeed, the novice speech pathologist who attempts to work with the hearing impaired may be chagrined to learn that all of his modern training could be counted as naught by the traditionalists unless he can "build the Yale Chart." The Yale or Northampton system is basically a phonetic system that attempts to use the English orthographic alphabet as a basis for phonetic spelling. Tables IX and X compare the Yale or Northampton symbols with those used by the International Phonetic Alphabet (IPA) and the common dictionary diacritical markings (often referred to as the Thorndike System in schools for the deaf).

The story behind the development of the Yale system is interesting. In the mid-1800s, Alexander Melville Bell developed a symbol system that he felt could be used to represent the speech

TABLE IX

PHONETIC CONSONANT SYMBOLS OF NORTHAMPTON, IPA, AND
DICTIONARY MARKINGS, WITH KEY WORDS

Primary Northampton Symbol	IPA Symbol	Dictionary Diacritical Markings	Key Words
h—	/h/	h	had, ahead
wh	/ʍ/	hw	when, everywhere
p	/p/	p	pie, sip, stopped
t	/t/	t	tie, sit, sitting
k	/k/	k	key, back, become
f	/f/	f	fan, leaf, coffee
th (1)	/θ/	th	thin, tooth, nothing
s (1)	/s/	s	see, makes, upset
sh	/ʃ/	sh	she, fish, sunshine
ch	/tʃ/	ch	chair, such, teacher
w—	/w/	w	we, awake
b	/b/	b	boy, cab, rabbit
d	/d/	d	day, mud, ladder
g	/g/	g	go, log, begged
v	/v/	v	vine, give, every
th (2)	/ð/	~~th~~	the, smooth, bother
z	/z/	z	zoo, size, lazy
zh	/ʒ/	zh	measure, vision
j	/dʒ/	j	jam, edge, enjoy
m	/m/	m	meat, team, camera
n	/n/	n	new, tin, any
ng	/ŋ/	ng	song, singer
l	/l/	l	low, bowl, color
r	/r/	r	red, bar, oral
y—	/j/	y	yes, canyon
x			box, taxi
qu	/kʍ/	kw	queen, liquid

Source: Donald R. Calvert and S. Richard Silverman, *Speech and Deafness,* 1975. Courtesy of The Alexander Graham Bell Association, Inc., Washington, D.C.

TABLE X

PHONETIC VOWEL SYMBOLS OF NORTHAMPTON, IPA, AND
DICTIONARY MARKINGS, WITH KEY WORDS

Primary Northampton Symbol	IPA Symbol	Dictionary Diacritical Markings	Key Words
1 oo 2	/u/	oo	boot, too
oo	/ʊ/	oo	book, could
aw	/ɔ/	o	awful, caught, law
ee	/i/	e	east, beet, be
-i-	/ɪ/	i	if, bit
-e-	/ɛ/	e	end, bet
-a-	/æ/	a	at, mat
a (r)	/a/	a (r)	odd, father, park
-u-	/ʌ/	u	up, cup
-u-	/ə/	ə	above, cobra
ur	/ɝ/	er	urn, burn, fur (General U.S.)
a-e	/eɪ/	a	able, made, may
i-e	/aɪ/	ī	ice, mice, my
oi	/ɔɪ/	oi	oil, coin, boy
u-e	/ju/	y͞oo	use, cute, few
o-e	/oʊ/	ō	old, boat, no

SOURCE: Donald R. Calvert and S. Richard Silverman, *Speech and Deafness*, 1975. Courtesy of The Alexander Graham Bell Association, Inc., Washington, D.C.

patterns of any language and to help foster a universal language. This symbol system, called visible speech, was based on the position of the articulators rather than a phonetic alphabet. The visible speech system was introduced to the Clark School for the Deaf in Northampton, Massachusetts, as an aid to teaching speech by Alexander Graham Bell, son of Alexander Melville. The history of Alexander Graham's contribution to science in general and to the hearing impaired in particular is well known.

The visible speech system was used as the basis for teaching speech at the Clark School (an oral program) until the 1880s. At that time Alice Worcester decided that the visible speech system, since it was based on symbols representing the position of the articulators for particular phonemes rather than an alphabet, was not providing any carry-over into reading. Worcester developed a phonetic alphabet that followed common English spelling as closely as possible. Some forty years later, Caroline Yale took the Worcester alphabet and arranged it in a more "logical" format and the result has come to be known as the Yale or Northampton Chart.

The Yale Chart is actually two charts, one for consonants and one for vowels. The consonants are arranged in columns and rows on the chart in such a manner that the phonemes in a particular column are related in manner of production (breath, voice, or nasal) and the phonemes in a specific row are related as to place of articulation (bilabials, linguadental, linguaalveolar, etc.). The vowels are arranged in a less specific manner, somewhat similar to the traditional vowel triangle. Placement of the vowels on the chart is made relative to vowel articulation: rounded vowels on one line, front vowels on another, dipthongs on another, etc.

The Yale Chart may originally have been conceived as a "logical" way of arranging a phonetic alphabet to show such relationships between phonemes as place and manner of articulation. However, it has evolved and been adopted as a system or framework for the entire program of speech education in many schools for the deaf. Traditionally, teachers in the lower grades begin "building the chart" by introducing, phoneme by phoneme, the consonants and vowels until, over the years, all of the phonemes and their interrelationships have been taught. Some teachers place such credance on the Yale charts that they use the phoneme order of the charts as a master phone development hierarchy and teach each phoneme in succession through the primary grades. Inherent in this entire process, of course, is the belief that speech is phonetic and composed of a series of independent phonemes, that independent phonemes can be taught, that a child can learn to take these phonemes and string them together to produce speech. The fallacy of such reasoning has been explained in previous chapters of this book and will be alluded to again in later portions of this chapter.

Of all the programs designed to develop speech in the hearing impaired, it is probable that none have been so blatant in promoting a phonetic or phoneme by phoneme approach as has the *McGinnis Association Method.* The Association Method, developed by Mildred McGinnis at the Central Institute for the Deaf, was intended for use with hearing impaired children who had failed to develop speech through more "normal" or "regular" teaching methods. Such children, often labeled *deaf-aphasic* or *deaf-learning disabled,* were assumed to belong to a special subgroup that required a particularly regimented curriculum and classroom atmosphere in order to develop speech. In this writer's experience, no other method of developing speech for the deaf has been so structured nor adhered to with as much dogmatic faith as the Association Method. The Method requires a sterile classroom with no visual distractions and strict attention to a repetitious teaching routine.

The Method begins with a specific set of commands such as "come," "stand on the line," "turn around," "sit down," etc. These commands are used in the classroom for the various stages of the Method. The Association Method breaks speech into subskills such as producing phonemes in isolation and combining phonemes into small phoneme clusters, phonemes into words, words into phrases, phrases into sentences, sentences into paragraphs, and paragraphs into stories. The teaching techniques — all of these stages rely heavily on rote memory — are very involved, laborious, and time-consuming; a description in detail of the Method is far beyond the scope of this chapter.

The Method is still used by some of the larger more traditionally oriented schools for the deaf. Most of these schools will have a teacher or teachers specially trained in the Association Method and the speech pathologist will usually not be expected to participate in the speech development activities. In some programs, however, the speech pathologist will be directly involved in the diagnostic and placement procedures and here caution must be urged. It should be understood that the Association Method was designed for use with aphasoid or language-learning disability like problems (LLD). While the speech pathologist may well want to ask whether or not the Method optimally meets the needs of deaf aphasic or LLD children (whatever these terms mean), he may also want to investigate the validity of the diagnostic procedures used to place children in the Method. In this writer's opinion, a deaf child's placement in a McGinnis Association Method classroom is often a product of tautological reasoning, i.e. the child is not learning speech because he is aphasic or LLD and he is aphasic or LLD because he cannot learn to speak.

In summary, most language development programs espouse a "natural approach" to communication development that makes little distinction between speech and language. This natural approach is based on the premise that experiences and concepts must precede speech. In practice, speech development programs and curricula are almost invariably phonetic in their approach. Usually it is assumed that the teaching of speech to the hearing impaired can be equated with the teaching of phonemes. Often, a phoneme development hierarchy forms the nucleus for the speech development program and this hierarchy is usually based on phoneme acquisition norms from hearing children, estimated relative ease of production or some "logical" format developed through face validity. Most, if not all, of these programs deviate drastically from modern linguistic findings and encourage the teaching of isolated phonemes and phonetic drill.

SPEECH PROBLEMS COMMON TO THE HEARING IMPAIRED

At the outset of this section, it should be stressed again that the hearing impaired population is far from homogeneous and factors such as type of hearing loss, extent of early training, type of early training, type and timing of amplification, etc., all contribute to variability in speaking ability. Even so, this writer's experience plus a review of the literature leads to the conclusion that, at least in some respects, indications of central tendencies can be found.

Since 1974, the Speech and Hearing Program at Lamar University has conducted a speech evaluation program for the Texas Education Agency. This process has resulted in speech diagnostic data on several hundred severely to profoundly hearing handicapped children. The following description of speech problems common to the deaf is based in large part on the results of experience rather than an extensive literature search. Moores (1978), Ling (1976), and especially Black (1971) and Nickerson (1975) have done a credible job of reviewing the literature on this issue and the reader is referred to these sources if documentation is desired. When evaluating the speech of the severe to profoundly hearing impaired, the staff at the Lamar University Speech and Hearing Center tend to focus their attention on the following areas: (a) oral examination, (b) articulation, (c) voice, (d) temporal factors, (e) nasality, (f) breathing patterns, (g) intelligibility, and (h) distracting habits. A description of each of these factors, some speculation as to possible causes, and a discussion of common remediation techniques follow.

Oral Examination

The speech pathologist has been trained to conduct oral examinations to assess structural capabilities for speech. The oral examination procedures used with a hearing impaired individual probably do not differ from those used with hearing subjects, but there are a few things that the speech pathologist should be aware.

Fraser (1971) estimates that about 50 percent of the profoundly deaf children are hearing impaired due to genetic factors: Konigsmark (1971) contends that there are at least seventy different types of hereditary deafness in man. Some of these types of hereditary deafness are coupled with varying degrees and combinations of facial and/or dental malformations that may or may not affect speech. In most of the larger schools for the deaf the speech pathologist can expect to find a few children with otocraniofacial syndromes, such as Treacher Collin's, Pierre Robin's Syndrome, Crouzon's Disease, Apert's Syndrome, etc., and children with deafness plus cleft palate are not unknown. In older deaf children and adults, the speech pathologist may find that surgical, orthodontic, and/or prosthetic work has been completed and the speech pathologist's role might be confined to helping the child learn to use existing structures. With younger children whose facial reconstruction process is not yet completed, the speech pathologist should be considered a part of the team that plans for surgery, orthodontia, prosthetic devices, and speech training.

The speech pathologist should pay particular attention to the teeth of the deaf child. In this writer's experience, dental caries and adventitious teeth in the hearing impaired are a serious problem. Where caries are concerned, it is probable that an oversolicitous home atmosphere is the causative factor in that little control of diet and dental hygiene is exercised. Indeed, at the Lamar University Summer Day School Program for the Hearing Impaired, the lunches packed for the children by their parents often consist solely of a soft drink, a candy bar, and a cupcake. At the same summer program, we have found the bulk of the children to have little knowledge of proper care of the teeth. This writer is not surprised to see severe dental caries in deaf children and has seen several cases where the teeth were reduced to blackened stubs. The problem of dental caries is mentioned here not so much because of a possible interference with speech but because the speech pathologist may be the professional in a position to make needed referrals. It would probably be wise for the speech pathologist to develop a referral list of dentists, orthodontists, pedodontists, etc., and to meet with these professionals to discuss the communication and health problems associated with hearing loss.

In the oral examination, the speech pathologist should look for adventitious teeth. Whether extra or misplaced teeth are more prevalent in the hearing handicapped is not known, but the author has found several cases where teeth needed to be removed because they actually interfered with speech. In two such cases, full sized molars were found growing from the center of the palatal vault. Here again it is the role of the speech pathologist to make referrals.

The writer has also seen several cases of muscular involvement of the articulators in deaf individuals and the speech pathologist should check the integrity of the sensorimotor system of the face, tongue, lips, etc.

Articulation

Previous chapters of this book have examined factors relating to articulation evaluation procedures and the subsequent remediation programming. The speech pathologist should be aware that such relatively recent concepts as deep testing for articulation, distinctive feature analysis, and distinctive feature therapy have not yet found wide acceptance in programs for the hearing impaired. Indeed, in most programs it is common for each child's school record to contain a yearly analysis of phoneme strengths and weaknesses stated in terms of distortion, omission, or substitution of particular phonemes in initial, medial, and final position. Often this traditional articulation analysis is the sole estimate of a child's speaking ability and yearly progress reports and teaching objectives are stated in terms of the articulation profile.

It is not uncommon to have a deaf child's annual speech evaluation consist of a list of problem phonemes with no mention of factors relating to voice, temporal factors, resonance problems, etc. In turn, speech objectives for a school year are often listed as four or five phonemes that, it is hoped, will be taught in the initial, medial, and final position. Similarly, term end reports of speech progress are often simply a listing of the few phonemes "mastered" during a specific time period. All this again points to the fact that in most speech programs for the hearing impaired, the emphasis and attention is on the phonetic aspects of individual phonemes. While this is probably indefensible in light of modern findings, the speech pathologist may have to be a master politician to effect any rapid meaningful changes.

In 1934, Hudgins published an often quoted report on the speech characteristics of the deaf and made several references to articulation. In the conclusion of the study, Hudgins lamented the fact that in general the speech of the hearing impaired was characterized by serious problems in all the variables he investigated. Hudgins hoped for a better future for speech for the deaf, which he felt would come through research and experience (Hudgins, 1934). It is this writer's opinion, however, if Hudgins could replicate his study of some half a century ago and use deaf children trained under "modern" methods he would find little, if any, differences. Nearly fifty years ago, Hudgins found the speech of the hearing impaired to be characterized by (a) slow temporal patterning, (b) inefficient use of the breath stream, (c) prolongation of vowels, (d) distortion of vowels, (e) abnormal rhythm, (f) excessive nasality, and (g) the addition of an undifferentiated neutral vowel between abutting consonants.

The present writer has found little reason to conclude that the speech of today's hearing impaired differs markedly from the deaf individuals studied by Hudgins so many years ago. Moores reaches this same conclusion and notes:

Given the lip service paid to the development of speech by all educators of the deaf and the dominance of the field by oral-only proponents until recent times, one might be inclined to expect that the teaching of speech to deaf children would be a well-researched, empirically based systematic process. Anyone so inclined would be sadly disappointed. With the exception of an excellent presentation of techniques used to develop speech at the Lexington School for the Deaf by Vorce (1974), and an overview of speech and deafness by Calvert and Silverman (1975), the contemporary literature is scarce. The situation in teaching speech to the deaf is analogous to that of the weather — everyone talks about it, but very few seem to do much about it. . . . Techniques and methods currently in use here have been in existence for fifty years or more. This, in itself, would not be a cause for alarm if there were evidence that the approaches had met with consistent success, but there is none. Although most programs view their approach to the teaching of speech as eclectic, a better description might be haphazard.

Working under the assumption that the first step to problem solving is to delineate the problem, this writer will, like Hudgins, discuss typical articulation problems of the deaf and hope that fifty years hence some writer does not decry the fact that we have made no progress in the past 100 years. The results of the speech evaluations at the Speech and Hearing Center at Lamar University indicate that the articulation of severe to profoundly hearing impaired individuals can be characterized by the following:

1. Excessive mandibular depression and movement.
2. Lack of tongue movement.
3. Posterior tongue positioning.
4. Voiced-voiceless confusions for consonants.
5. Problems with coarticulation.
6. Substitution of visible sounds for those difficult to see.
7. Better articulation for phonemes occurring at the beginning of words than for those in the medial or final position.
8. An interaction between type of hearing loss and the

acoustic characteristics of phonemes in that the hearing impaired usually have more articulation problems with high frequency sounds such as sibilants.

9. Stop/plosive confusion and the intrusion of an undifferentiated neutral vowel between abutting consonants.

It is probable that the excessive mandibular depression is at least in part related to teaching methods. In the phoneme by phoneme teaching technique, it is common for the teacher, in an effort to provide visual cues, to speak with exaggerated mouth opening and jaw movement. Often such "tongue reading" may be accompanied by mirror work with the teacher and child seated in front of a mirror so that the child can compare his articulatory movements with those of the speech pathologist/ teacher. While this technique is not inherently harmful, it does contribute to excessive mandibular depression if the teacher or speech pathologist fails to teach the child to produce the phoneme with normal articulation once the exaggerated target has been reached. It should be obvious that exaggerated jaw opening is interrelated with abnormal coarticulation, temporal patterns, resonance, etc.

In analyzing the articulation of the deaf via spectrography, this writer has found, as did Black (1971), that the second formant is relatively stationary. The reader is reminded that the second formant responds to changes in the position of the articulators, especially tongue position in vowels and vowellike voiced consonants. A stationary second formant is usually attributed to a lack of tongue motion. This writer has found that the tongue of the deaf is often retracted to the rear of the mouth where it remains with little or no mobility during the act of speaking. When this occurs, the jaws and lips are used to try to articulate the various speech sounds but the results, as would be expected, are poor. This writer is unaware of any objective data that indicates why the hearing impaired tend to speak with a retracted and relatively motionless tongue, but Drum (1963), who is himself deaf, has speculated that it is caused by a self-conscious effort to "swallow" the voice or to put the act of speaking deeper in the throat where vibrations can be felt more readily. This writer wonders, however, if the retracted tongue is not more related to the exaggerated mandibular depression already mentioned. That is, it is possible that with a depressed mandible the "natural" position of the tongue is to the posterior portion of the oral cavity. Whatever the cause, the speech pathologist would do well to watch for the problem since a retracted tongue is obviously related to problems of resonance, articulation, and temporal patterning.

Teachers of the deaf have long battled with the problem of voiced-voiceless confusions and many traditional speech teaching techniques are designed to lessen the problem. In the evaluation of the hearing impaired person's speech, the speech pathologist will often make note of the voice-voiceless confusions and then list as a major objective the amelioration of the problem. While tactual sensation (child's hand to speech pathologist's throat) or visual feedback (oscilloscope) are often recommendations made for treatment, it should be remembered that programming for speech and coarticulation are extremely rapid processes. While it may be possible to help a child differentiate between voiced and voiceless sounds when these sounds are isolated, it is usually much more difficult to remove the problem from ongoing speech.

Teachers of the hearing handicapped are often plagued by the fact that a child can produce all of the elements of a word but cannot produce the word as a unit. The speech pathologist will often find this to be true during a speech evaluation session. For example, a child may be able to produce an /s/, a /t/, an /r/, an /i/, and another /t/, but be unable to coordinate these phonemes into a coarticulated "strit." It is felt that such a problem in coarticulation is evident in all age groups and accounts in large part for the low level of intelligibility of deaf speech. The speech pathologist may well attribute problems related to coarticulation to the prevalent practice of teaching phonemes in isolation and the concentration of teaching time on phonemes rather than phoneme combinations in words and phrases.

A speech pathologist who looks for trends within the array of articulatory problems encountered will often note that the deaf person is not making random articulatory errors, but rather is using some pattern or phonemic rule that differs from that used by the hearing population. This is perhaps most evident with those individuals who consistently substitute visible sounds for those difficult to see. Such a pattern has been recognized for some time and several writers have hypothesized that the better articulation for the more visable phonemes is a positive indication of the utility of visual feedback as a teaching/correction tool. From this assumption has come several visual speech aids. These visual speech aids have ranged in complexity from simple feather boards used to indicate nasal air flow to complicated electronic filter analyzers that indicate changing format positions with light indicators (Pickett, 1971). While a few of these visual speech aids have served a dual purpose and have been used as evaluative/diagnostic instruments, their main utility has traditionally been as a teaching/correction tool.

Another recurring pattern is for phonemes to be more correctly produced at the beginning of a word than in other positions. This is probably due to the fact that the effects of coarticulatory feedback are less for the initial position. It should be remembered that in the speech of the "normal" hearing person, neither phonemes nor words are spoken in isolation and the concept of the initial phoneme position may have little practical utility because of backward and forward coarticulation effects experienced in varying linguistic environments. With the hearing impaired, however, a choppy or broken word by word rhythm pattern is often encountered and, therefore, the initial position often becomes "easier" than the medial and final.

The speech pathologist will often find that a neutral vowel has been added between abutting consonants by the hearing impaired. Thus, in the word *captain*, a schwa might often be inserted between the /p/ and /t/. In this writer's experience, this phenomenon can usually be attributed to a phoneme by phoneme teaching approach that fails to make a distinction between stops and plosives and that encourages the use of excessive amounts of breath pressure for plosives. It is a common practice for teachers to indicate the release of breath pressure for plosives by blowing out candles or by causing feathers or bits of tissue paper to scatter with the release of breath pressure. Such practices are often *not* followed by teaching techniques designed to contrast the plosive with the stop and the deaf child then produces all stop/plosives in an aspirated, released manner. Aside from that, it should also be mentioned that the amount of breath pressure needed to blow out candles, scatter feathers, and knock over a tissue held in the hand far exceeds the breath pressure used in the normal articulation of plosives.

Voice

The voice of the deaf is usually characterized by problems relating to fundamental frequency and vocal attack. These two factors will be covered separately here, but it should be stressed that they are in fact interrelated. Two additional factors, intensity and duration, will also be discussed.

Since most hearing impaired individuals have some hearing in the low frequencies and since the fundamental frequency of normal speakers is low relative to the other components of the complex speech wave, it is often assumed that at least the fundamental of the deaf should be normal or nearly so. Ling and Ling (1978) go so far as to say that if young deaf children " . . . have useful residual hearing and are fitted with appropriate hearing aids at this stage, natural voice quality and variation of voice patterns can usually be preserved without specific auditory or speech training." However, if the speech pathologist could travel to the various educational programs for the deaf across the nation and sample the voice characteristics of children, teenagers, and young adults, he would find but few with "normal" vocal patterns. Whether this should be attributed to the hearing loss or to teaching practices or both remains to be seen.

Most writers discussing the voice of the deaf pay the bulk of their attention to the fact that a high fundamental occurs so often. While this is no doubt true, this writer has found frequency related problems at both ends of the spectrum. The speech pathologist will not often find a deaf person with an abnormally low voice, but it does occur. At present, we have little definitive information with which to specify the causative factors of fundamentals that are either too high or too low. Drum (1963) suggests that vibratory feedback from a low voice may reinforce the use of the low fundamental but no hard data were presented.

If Drum is correct, one must wonder why a low fundamental among the deaf is relatively rare. It has been suggested that the high fundamental that one hears so often with the hearing impaired may be attributed to an underdeveloped larynx (Holm, 1970).

It is felt by some writers that the laryngeal musculature of the deaf is underdeveloped because of a relative lack of use (Black, 1971). That is, compared to hearing people, the deaf tend to speak less often and, therefore, supposedly use the larynx less often, which is thought to lead to a lack of "laryngeal exercise." This lack of exercise is thought to preclude normal growth of the laryngeal structures and the resulting relatively small vocal apparatus produces a high fundamental. The fallacy of such a notion is no doubt obvious to the speech pathologist but the idea is so pervasive in deaf education that some discussion is warranted.

It must be remembered that the primary functions of the structures used for speech are *not* speech: speech is an overlaid function. The tongue was "designed" to move food, the soft palate was "designed" to close off the velopharyngeal port during swallowing and sucking, the lungs were "designed" for gaseous exchange, etc. and the exercise that these structures get in performing their primary function is sufficient for muscular development. Speech curricula for the hearing impaired, however, usually contain exercises for the lips, jaws, tongue, soft palate, etc. and many teachers of the deaf begin their daily speech lessons with "articulatory gymnastics." That such activities are unnecessary and a waste of time should be obvious.

This writer was once approached by a graduate student from physical education who wanted him to serve on her dissertation committee. The topic of her dissertation concerned the development of exercises designed to increase the lung capacity of the deaf. When she was asked why such exercises were needed, she explained that it was obvious that, since the deaf spoke but rarely, they used their lungs less often than did hearing people and, therefore, their lungs were underdeveloped. After it was explained to her that the primary purpose of the respiratory system was not breath support for speaking and that deaf children exercised their lungs when they ran, played, walked, etc., she wondered why she had been allowed by the other members of her graduate committee to progress so far on her project — she had written the first two chapters of her dissertation without finding a reference or a professional who found fault with her reasoning.

The larynx, of course, was "designed" primarily for protective functions and receives sufficient exercise in performing these primary functions. This writer has talked to several otolaryngologists concerning this issue and all of them see no reason to assume that the larynx of the hearing impaired should not be normal and none of them report finding a deaf child with an underdeveloped larynx. Hard data, however, are not available.

The speech pathologist will often find *laryngeal tension* accompanying a high fundamental frequency and it is felt that a cause and effect relationship exists between these two variables. This writer has long been convinced that several speech therapy practices traditionally used with the deaf contribute to laryngeal tension and that this tension results in a higher vocal tone. Often such tension is related to the attitude that speech is a difficult task but that success could be achieved if the deaf child would only *try harder*. It is possible too that some therapy techniques such as those designed to increase phonation duration time or words per breath group may be directly related to laryngeal tension but again no hard data are available. Suffice it to say that the speech pathologist should look for evidence of laryngeal tension during the initial examination and then be cautious of therapy or advice that could lead to tension.

Some evidence exists that indirectly indicates that the higher fundamental found in the deaf population is probably functional rather than organic in nature. Holbrook and Crawford (1970) describe a behavior modification program that has had good results in training the deaf to bring their high fundamentals down to within more normal limits. If the high fundamentals of Holbrook and Crawford's subjects had been related to an organic factor such as underdeveloped laryngeal structures, it is doubtful that the fundamentals could have been lowered with the rapidity and ease reported by the researchers.

Holbrook and Crawford's technique consisted of giving visual feedback relative to the fundamental through a modified pitch meter. It is interesting to note that though Holbrook and Crawford report excellent results in using an electronic visual display to correct an abnormally high fundamental or nasal resonance, Ling and Ling (1978) caution against the use of electronic visual displays because their use could cause the child to rely less on residual hearing. Ling and Ling (1978) state that " . . . no visual display or cue system can as effectively supplement speechreading as does residual hearing and that to employ them with children who have useful residual hearing may hinder their use of audition."

The speech pathologist has been taught in classes on voice disorders that all individuals have one fundamental which would be considered optimal for that person's age, sex, size, weight, etc. The speech pathologist has also been taught to make judgments relative to a person's habitual fundamental and to decide whether or not a discrepancy exists between an individual's habitual and optimal fundamentals. Of course, the trick is the determination of the optimal and the habitual fundamentals. Some clinicians find the habitual pitch by listening to a speech sample and using a pitch pipe, a piano, or a "perfect ear" to determine the average pitch used. This habitual pitch is then contrasted with the optimal pitch. The optimal pitch is usually determined through some formula that uses fractions of the individual's pitch range such as one-third of the way up from the lowest to the highest pitch. Since many deaf children and adults exhibit a limited pitch range it is usually difficult to determine with any degree of accuracy their optimal pitch. It has traditionally been believed that a deaf person's laugh corresponds to his optimal pitch since laughing is a "relaxed and natural act." Whether or not there is any truth to this bit of folklore is unknown. In practice, if the fundamental of a deaf person is within the range of normal, the speech pathologist should not be too concerned that a slight variation between optimal and habitual pitch might exist.

The speech pattern of the deaf is often said to contain little variation in fundamental frequency between and within utterances. Such a monotone approach to speaking is a problem with which the speech pathologist should be concerned and evidence of monotone should be noted in the initial examination. This writer has seen, however, abrupt pitch changes that habitually occur at particular parts of a sentence (pitch stereotypes), frequently at the end of sentences. For example, the writer once worked with a teenage deaf girl who habitually spoke all the words of a sentence with an average of about 300 Hz but usually raised the fundamental of the last word to above 500 Hz. Such monotone or stereotyped pitch patterns may be distracting to the listener and deserve remedial attention.

In some hearing impaired individuals a *breathy voice quality* may be discerned. That is, the art of approximating the vocal folds is often inefficient and more air than is needed for phonation is used. Such an aspirate voice quality typically lacks volume and is unpleasant to hear. In addition, the inefficient use of the air stream necessitates a more frequent inhalation pattern that in turn interferes with temporal patterning and shortens the phonation duration time. That is, the deaf individual is often unable to sustain phonation for longer than a few seconds.

The fact that the deaf often have a problem with phonation duration does not mean that the speech pathologist should begin recommending wholesale duration exercises. It should be remembered that problems in sustaining phonation are symptomatic, not causative, and that exercises designed to increase phonation duration can and do lead to vocal tension. The writer has often seen teachers of the deaf leading their students through exercises in which the duration of particular vowels were timed. The problem with such an exercise is that the children and teacher can get carried away to the point that the children are pushing and straining during the last few seconds of phonation. Such strain and tension can only contribute to the speech problems of the deaf. The speech pathologist or teacher of the deaf should probably spend more time helping the hearing impaired individual achieve an efficient phonation pattern and less time on phonation duration drills.

Volume is also a problem for the hearing impaired. As noted, the breathy voice quality often contributes to this problem.

Another factor, nasal resonance, often adds to the problem in that vocal intensity is decreased when the nasal chamber is coupled with the oral chamber (Curtis, 1968). Additionally, the deaf have a difficult time adjusting their intensity to background conditions. In a noisy situation (in a crowd, in a car, etc.) the voice of the deaf person may not carry well enough to be heard. By the same token, the deaf are often embarrassed to learn that in a quiet situation, such as in church, their voice has travelled much further than they had intended. The speech pathologist would do well in the initial examination to check for volume control and range and, if needed, to develop later lessons aimed at helping the hearing impaired with this problem.

This writer has often had speech pathologists ask him if the hearing impaired population develops laryngeal polyps, nodules, contact ulcers, or other symptoms of vocal abuse. The reasoning behind the question is sound in that in the hearing population we would expect such factors as compensatory laryngeal tension and an inappropriate fundamental pitch level to result in laryngeal pathology. The writer has never been able to adequately answer this excellent question and can only say that he has not found any references in the literature that have been of any help and that research is needed. Perhaps this research can best be started by the speech pathologist who works with the deaf and who makes referrals of suspected voice cases. At present, it is all too probable that any symptoms of vocal abuse are attributed to the hearing loss and polyps, nodules and contact ulcers go undetected.

Temporal Factors

Temporal problems are evident in both the segmental and the suprasegmental aspects of the speech of the hearing impaired. As previously noted, the phoneme production rate is often (if not usually) slower than normal. Vowels particularly are elongated. The writer has found through spectrographic analysis that vowels of the deaf are often four to six times longer in duration. This elongation of phonemes plus problems with coarticulation imparts a slow, labored, and choppy flavor to the segmental factors of deaf speech. On the suprasegmental level, we often find that juncture problems related to grouping words within breath units and not knowing when to pause interact with the above mentioned segmental problems to produce a speech rhythm that is vastly different from the temporal patterning used by hearing people.

Some educators of the deaf have realized that rhythmic factors are a problem in the speech of the hearing impaired and attempts have been made to alleviate the problem. Some programs, however, have decided that a poor sense of rhythm leads to poor speech. That is, it is sometimes assumed that temporal factors are the cause, rather than the effect of poor speech habits. From this assumption, only a small mental step is needed to arrive at the conclusion that teaching body rhythm to deaf preschoolers and primary-aged children will give the youngsters a sense of timing upon which later speech can be built. This writer is aware of at least two large residential schools that, until recently, appeared to place more emphasis on what they called *eurhythmics* than on actual practice with conversational speech. Under such a program, activities during the early years were concentrated on marching to varying drum beats, learning dance steps, "listening" to music, feeling the vibrations of pianos, learning rhythmic body movements, etc. Supposedly, the children should learn in later years to use their hard earned sense of rhythm as a carrier for speech patterns. It seems to this writer that a deaf child with a good sense of rhythm (whatever that means) can still have temporarily related speech problems if factors such as faulty juncture, disturbed coarticulation and a word by word approach to sentences are present.

Some programs stress the teaching of a more normal speech rhythm through various combinations of TVAK (tactual, visual, auditory, kinesthetic) feedback. The tactual sense has been used to some degree through tapping speech rhythm on a child's arm or by having a child hold a vibrator that responds to speech rhythm. Several visual displays such as the oscilloscope and the video articulator have been used (Bargstadt, Hutchinson, and Nerbonne, 1978). The kinesthestic sense usually is considered to provide information relative to phoneme production but some programs have stressed that kinesthesia can also give feedback relative to rhythm. There is a relatively new school of thought that places primary emphasis on residual hearing and attempts to lessen the impact of reliance on any sense other than hearing. This is most evident in the work of Ling and Ling (1978) who propose that only those with no useful residual audition be introduced to any feedback system other than hearing.

Nasality

For discussion of nasal resonance, it is important that the speech pathologist keep in mind that hypernasality is often as much in the mind of the listener as it is in the nose of the speaker. That is, it would appear that factors other than an inadequate velopharyngeal closure can contribute to the perception of nasality. For instance, we know that if we take a recording of a normal speaker judged to have no nasality problems and mechanically alter the rate or rhythm or both, the recording may then be judged to be more nasal. The speech pathologist working with the cleft palate case has used this principle to help alleviate the effects of velopharyngeal valving problems and the same idea can be used in speech remediation for the hearing impaired. In fact, as we shall see later, most of the techniques used with the cleft palate case can be readily adapted to the deaf individual.

Nasal resonance is a major problem in the speech for the deaf. This resonance problem is nearly always at the hyper rather than at the hypo end of the nasal resonance spectrum. The hearing impaired person often speaks with the velopharyngeal port open at all times or opens and closes the port in a nearly random manner. Teachers of the deaf have been battling the problem of nasality since the beginning of the profession and a number of techniques have evolved. Most of them, however, do not fare well when compared with what we know of speech physiology and perception.

Some teachers of the deaf either confuse nasal air emission with nasal resonance or do not understand velopharyngeal valving or both. The writer has seen teachers have children hold their nares closed with their fingers while speaking in an effort to help the child learn not to "talk through the nose." One teacher required some of her children to wear a clothespin on the nose during the speech lessons. The writer has known of teachers of the deaf who confused the gag reflex with velopharyngeal closure. In one instance, a teacher laid a child on his back on a table, had the child open his mouth and say "ahhh" while she dropped Cheerios® onto the back wall of the pharynx in an effort to make the child gag so that he could be "taught" how to close off the velopharyngeal port. Other teachers who have been confused as to the role of the gag reflex in speech have used tongue depressors to initiate the gag. Such practices, thankfully, are not widespread but the speech pathologist should be aware that misconceptions concerning the cause of nasal resonance problems do exist and he may have to conduct considerable inservice on the topic.

As mentioned earlier, many teachers of the deaf assume that at least some of the speech problems of the hearing impaired are caused by underdeveloped articulatory musculature. This is quite evident in a number of programs that stress exercises for "strengthening the soft palate." In most cases these exercises entail sucking and blowing but some programs also contain phonetic drills designed to contrast nasal and nonnasal sounds and thus make the soft palate stronger. In 1967, an international conference of oral educators of the deaf was held and the papers from this conference have been published (Volta Bureau, 1967). In reading the various reports presented at the conference, one is struck by how often reference is made of the "need" for palatal exercises. Hyde and Engle (1977) are also apparently of the opinion that (1) nasal resonance problems of the deaf are related to a weak or uncontrolled soft palate and (2) that blowing the nose can strengthen the soft palate and/or bring it under control. In their speech curriculum, they specify how the nose should be blown ("open mouth, breath in, shut lips, hold breath, blow, wipe") and caution the teacher or speech clinician to "wipe the nose with a tissue every time the activity is attempted."

Another pervasive misconception that the speech pathologist will have to contend with is that a knowledge of anatomy and physiology will help in speech production. The writer observed one group of high school-aged deaf children who could draw and label all of the skeletal, muscular, and nerve components of the head and neck. In the case of nasality, it is typical for a teacher of the deaf to spend considerable time with visual displays and models showing how the soft palate, faucial pillars, and back wall of the pharynx work to close the velopharyngeal port.

It may well be up to the speech pathologist to provide information relative to the fact that the speed of articulatory programming would preclude conscious control of velopharyngeal valving *even* if it were not true that the structures that act to close the velopharyngeal port possess little sensory nerve endings with which to provide feedback relative to muscular movement.

Once the speech pathologist has explained the futility of palatal exercises and lessons designed to bring velopharyngeal closure under conscious control, he will be asked "what does work?" It is at this point that the speech pathologist can describe the speech habilitation techniques used with the cleft palate population. In this writer's experience, teachers of the deaf have welcomed such suggestions as (a) making light quick contact for plosives, (b) changing habitual pitch level, (c) increasing the speaking rate, and (d) being certain that the tongue is not retracted to the rear of the oral cavity.

Breathing Patterns

In the 1930s, Hudgins and Scuri both described the breathing patterns used by the deaf while speaking (Hudgins, 1934, 1936, 1937; and Scuri, 1935). These early writers note that the deaf tend to use more exhaled breath while speaking than do hearing speakers. Commenting on this, Nickerson (1975) states that the increased air flow during speaking causes the deaf to interrupt the rhythm pattern and thus contributes to the temporal problems already discussed. Nickerson (1975) also notes that, compared to hearing speakers, the deaf tend to expel much more breath while speaking and " . . . consequently they are likely to interrupt the speech flow more frequently in order to permit the intake of air." This constant interruption of the speech pattern has obvious negative effects on the rhythm pattern. Note too that Nickerson states that the deaf speaker is likely to use more breath while speaking than while not speaking. That is, the amount of air exchanged is increased over time as the deaf person speaks. For the hearing speaker, this is not the case. This increase in amount of air can and does lead to the discomfort of hyperventilation among some deaf persons while speaking. The writer was told by one deaf adult that she became dizzy and felt "light headed" whenever she spoke for any length of time. How widespread this problem is, the writer does not know, but it could in part explain why many deaf people are reluctant to speak.

Scuri (1935), Hudgins (1934), and Nickerson (1975) are all of the opinion that the breathing problems of the deaf are in large part related to *inefficient vocal attack*. That is, the deaf tend to approximate the vocal folds incompletely and a significant amount of breath is wasted during phonation. This uneconomical use of the breath stream in turn leads to a lessening of the number of words possible per breath. It is not uncommon to find a deaf child who cannot produce more than one or two words before taking another breath. In trying to combat this problem, many teachers of the deaf appear to be concentrating on the symptom rather than the cause. That is, emphasis is placed on drills designed to increase the number of words produced per breath group rather than to improve the efficiency of the vocal fold approximation. In this writer's experience, drills designed to increase words per breath group without a concomitant emphasis on proper phonation often lead to further speech problems. For instance, a deaf person may learn that by increasing the amount of air inhaled, more words can be spoken per breath group. This abnormally large inhalation phase is often distractingly audible and may add to the hyperventilation and rhythm problems already discussed. Also, if the child pushes and strains at the end of the breath group to get that one last word out, the added tension can lead to problems such as an increased fundamental.

Intelligibility

Studies of speech intelligibility consistently indicate that, at best, naive listeners can be expected to understand only 20 to 25 percent of the speech of the deaf (Smith, 1973; Markides, 1970; Heidinger, 1972; Ling, 1976). This is plausible in light of the numerous speech problems. The speech pathologist should try to get some estimate of the speech intelligibility of the deaf individuals with whom he is involved. This estimate may be as informal as engaging the deaf person in conversation or as formal as taking speech sample recordings and playing them to naive audiences. The writer knows of at least one residential school for the deaf where annual recordings are made to play before naive high school-aged listeners. These resulting intelligibility scores are then used as an estimate of speech progress.

Distracting Habits

The speech pathologist will often find that the deaf individual may engage in any number of distracting habits that interfere with speaking. These habits may include audible breathing, popping noises made with the lips, facial grimaces, etc. The speech pathologist may find that helping the deaf individual correct these problems is very difficult. The writer remembers working with a very bright deaf preschooler who consistently made popping noises with her lips while speaking. The writer lost track of this girl for some twelve years, only to later find that the popping sounds were still a part of the girl's verbal behavior. The popping noises were so distracting that it is most probable that the girl's teachers and speech pathologists had tried to help her stop making the noises. The difficulty of removing such habits will be appreciated by the speech pathologist who has worked with such functional speech disorders.

Summary

The above section may best be summarized by a short sentence written by John Black (1971): "The speech of deaf children differs from normal speech in all regards." We have seen that the speech pathologist needs to be aware of common problems relating to voice, articulation, rhythm, respiration, and resonance. While some of these problems can be attributed to the hearing loss, many may also be directly related to teaching practices. Rather than being depressed about the fact that faulty education/habilitation practices have historically contributed to the speech problems of the deaf, the speech pathologist should feel encouraged. Teachers of the deaf are in the main intelligent, hard-working, caring individuals. This writer has found them to be open for suggestions as to how to improve the speech of the deaf. It is probable that these suggestions will have to come from the speech pathologist who understands not only his profession, but also how to work within a system to bring about change.

A BETTER CABIN?

The writer's father once told him not to tear down his shack until he could build a better cabin. In all honesty, it is tempting to disregard this sage advice and end this chapter at this point. It has been relatively easy to delineate the common problems associated with speech development and correction. It is going to be much more difficult to "build a better cabin" by specifying an improved framework for helping the deaf individual develop and improve his speech. Further, as suggested in Chapter 6, research data relative to the comparative efficacy of selected approaches are not available. However, in light of the apparent dismal failure of many of the traditional approaches taken in the past and based on our current knowledge of speech and the hearing impaired child, the following suggestions appear to be warranted. They should be subjected to clinical trial by clinicians and, where possible, should be empirically tested.

Premise I

Speech correction and speech development are not equivalent and should not be treated as such by parents, teachers, and speech pathologists. All too often, parents and teachers assume that the way to develop speech in the deaf is to "teach" each phoneme and then to correct any errors that arise. Such an approach has proven to be inefficient and to depart drastically from normal speech development. Modern writers are calling for better auditory management of young hearing impaired children such that residual hearing can aid in a more normal speech development (Ross and Giolas, 1978). Others are also calling for better utilization of compensatory feedback systems such as kinesthesia and touch (Ling and Ling, 1978). Some writers appear to be convinced that speech, if it is to develop at all, will appear as a natural outgrowth of language development and that the best stimulus to both language and speech is manual communication (Moores, 1978). In this writer's opinion, speech *and* language development should be the goals of the early

preschool and elementary school years and didactic speech remediation techniques should be withheld until the child has
enough language to cooperate in and understand the speech
remediation program. This should not be interpreted as
suggesting that the speech pathologist should not work with the
deaf child until he is older. On the contrary, the speech
pathologist should play a vital role in helping the young child to
develop speech and language skills.

Premise II

Parental involvement in speech development is to be encouraged and directed but *realistic* goals must be stressed. The speech
pathologist would do well to speculate on the personal and
family trauma that is inherent in the discovery that one's child is
deaf. All too often, parents and family members focus on the
most apparent symptom of the hearing loss and their major
concern is "will the baby ever talk?" Eugene Mindel, a psychia-
trist who has worked with many families that have a deaf child,
feels that this early focus on speech may in many cases be the first
symptom of a denial of the handicap (Mindel, 1971). That is,
some families reach the conclusion that their child will not "really" be deaf if he can talk. Mindel notes that "parents should be
protected against developing beliefs that early intervention can
accomplish the task of having their child, especially a profoundly
deaf child, function as a normal child." To fail to do so may allow
or encourage the family to place undue emphasis on speech with
a concomitant lack of emphasis on personal, social, academic and
language development. Along this same line, Moores (1978)
states:

> Finally, in their desire for the child to be an extension of themselves,
> parents ask, "Will our child be normal? Above all, will speech be possi-
> ble?" It is at this point that professionals first fail deaf children and their
> families. If parents receive inaccurate and misleading advice at this
> time, the negative effects may never be overcome. It is only natural for
> parents to think that the basic problem of the deaf child is an inability to
> speak, when, in reality, the basic problem is in inability to hear. Profes-
> sionals have the responsibility to ensure that — as gently as possible, but
> also as firmly as possible — parents are made to understand this.

The speech pathologist should also consider that a sense of
guilt often accompanies the discovery of deafness. Parents often

feel that their child is being punished for real or imagined "sins" of the parents. Mindel says that "after discovery of deafness, the parents may attempt to assuage their guilt through overcompensation. . . . " Frequently parents are told in early counseling sessions that their child will develop good speech if the *parents try hard enough.* The writer has often seen parents accept this advice and expend superhuman efforts to help improve the child's speech. Parents have paid for daily speech therapy, hired live-in speech tutors for full-time help, and, in general, made speech for their deaf child the central focus for the entire family. The writer is acquainted with one mother who for a twenty-year period made a daily round trip of 150 miles for speech correction for her child and structured the home atmosphere to resemble a continuous speech therapy session. All too often, however, the child fails to achieve the speech-related goals set by the parents. When this happens the parents may conclude that they did not try hard enough, that the child did not try hard enough, and/or that they were originally given bad advice. Moores (1978) also discusses this issue in a cogent statement:

> Some organizations in the field of deafness function primarily to facilitate the development of speech in deaf children. This is a commendable undertaking, but certainly not the only — or even the most important — goal for young deaf children. One can only guess how many thousands of families have been harmed by the counseling of well-meaning but misinformed individuals whose advice has not really been aimed at the healthy development of the deaf child but rather at the neurotic selfish needs of parents who want their children, as psychological and physical extensions of themselves, to be "normal," that is, speaking. Mindel and Vernon (1972) make the point, and the present author agrees, that the fixation on normalcy (speaking) prevents parents from working through their grief to the mature acceptance of deafness that is a prerequisite for adequate psychological and social development. Without such acceptance, parents will not develop healthy mechanisms to cope with the outer reality of a child with a hearing loss and the inner reality of adjusting to the feeling of loss of a desired normal child.

In a good educational program, the speech pathologist will be called on to answer the parent's questions relating to speech development. Parents should be informed that not all deaf people develop useful speech and that, at present, we find it difficult, if not impossible, to prognosticate, especially with the very young deaf child. Parents should be urged to help in speech development, but they should be carefully counseled such that the deaf child is accepted as an individual with potential in areas in addition to speech such as language development, personality development, social skills, academic achievement, etc.

This writer has often found it helpful to have a member of the adult deaf community speak to parents concerning speech development. Many adult deaf people have good speech skills and a healthy attitude toward all forms of communication. A telling statement from one of the author's adult deaf friends comes to mind: "If you want to help us with our speech so that we can better communicate with hearing people when we want to, fine; but if you want to help us with our speech so that we can become imitation hearing people, forget it."

Premise III

At present, not all deaf individuals develop functional speech and there may be a point at which further efforts to develop speech for a particular child are not economical in terms of time and effort. The reader may well wonder why the writer lists such a statement as a somewhat novel premise when research has repeatedly shown that average speech intelligibility at schools for the deaf in the United States is no better than 20 percent for words in sentences and that the speech of many deaf people is so unintelligible as to preclude any but the most rudimentary utility. The reason for including this "The Emperor has no clothes!" premise should become clear with the following example.

The writer was asked to serve as a consultant to an educational program for the deaf and to make recommendations concerning the speech clinician's role. The writer found that the speech clinician was providing therapy to sixty deaf children on an individual and small group basis. Because she was attempting to spread her services equally among sixty children, each child received but a few minutes of help each week. The advice given by the writer to the school administrators was that their speech pathologist's time was not being used efficiently. Options open to them appeared to be (a) hire additional speech pathologists, (b) determine which children were good candidates for speech therapy and allow the speech clinician to concentrate her efforts where they would do the most good, or (c) put the speech clinician in an advisory role to the classroom teachers and let the teachers do the actual speech therapy.

The school administrators were reluctant to adopt any of the options. The hiring of additional speech pathologists was not deemed possible due to budgetary restrictions. The administrators liked the idea of concentrating the speech pathologist's efforts on the "good speech candidates" but they were extremely nervous about the reactions of parents whose children would be labeled as "poor speech risks." The administrators would have agreed to changing the role of the speech clinician to that of advisor were it not for the fact that the speech clinician had only recently been hired and that the position had been created because of parental pressure. The parents were convinced that a speech pathologist was an expert who could improve their children's speech and had prevailed on the school administration to create the position. Each parent was convinced of the wonderful powers of the speech clinician and each wanted their child to have his fair share of the clinician's time. The entire situation would have been different if the parents had been given earlier counsel regarding the fact that not all deaf people develop speech and that the time may come when to continue to try to improve speech can only frustrate the child and consume time better spent on endeavors where the child has a greater chance of success.

Inherent in Premise III is some form of prognostic or evaluative procedure. That is, how does one decide who will and who will not benefit from the speech clinician's time? The writer does not have in mind the classifying of youngsters into "speech" and "no speech" groups at the preschool or even the elementary level. Rather, he is concerned with those children, fourteen and fifteen years old who have little usable speech and who have shown little, if any, speech improvement for several years. In this writer's experience, such children can, through concentrated efforts, still receive some benefit from speech therapy but this improvement costs dearly in time and effort and these commodities are often better spent in other areas for the deaf teenager.

A diagnostic procedure may already be available to help the speech clinician in determining who would be a good "speech risk." This evaluation technique is based on the premise that the way in which an individual codes his language can affect his speech production. Perhaps the leading proponent of this tenet has been R. Conrad. It has long been supposed that in the hearing population we process, retrieve, and store our language related activities in a code that is acoustic or speech motor in nature (Locke, 1970). Using a short term memory (STM) task, Conrad (1970, 1973) was able to separate deaf subjects into two groups, those who coded language in acoustic or speech motor fashion and those who did not. Interestingly, Conrad found that those who coded language related material in a manner similar to hearing people (acoustic or speech motor) had developed speech that was superior to the group that coded language in means other than acoustic or speech motor factors. Thus by the result of a STM paper and pencil task, Conrad was able to predict the relative speech skills of deaf children. How good the Conrad technique would be as a prognostic tool and at what age coding strategies become "set" and difficult to change remains to be seen, but the work of Conrad is a big step in the right direction.

The manner in which language related material is coded by the deaf plays a major role in determining the quality of speech production. It should be stressed that while hearing people use a mediation process based on acoustic or speech motor features, the deaf individual has the option of using alternatives such as speechreading, fingerspelling, sign language, semantic factors, etc. Moulton and Beasley (1975) discuss these coding options and present a STM instrument designed to evaluate the relative strengths of semantic and sign language coding. The point of all this is that since Conrad has shown that a lack of acoustic or speech motor mediation in the deaf is usually accompanied by relatively poor speech skills, and since Conrad and Moulton and Beasley have specified ways in which the coding strategies of the deaf may be determined, it may now be possible to evaluate the efficacy of different teaching strategies and to begin to make better prognostic statements concerning the speech of the deaf.

The reader is cautioned against reaching the conclusion that the findings of Conrad and of Moulton and Beasley indicate that coding by sign and coding by acoustic or speech motor features are mutually exclusive and that only through a singular coding strategy (acoustic or speech motor) is functional speech possible. Such a conclusion quickly leads to the assumption that a total communication educational program precludes good speech because it fosters mediation strategies other than acoustic or speech motor. It must be remembered that the philosophy of total communication calls for the use of any and all forms of communication such as speech, fingerspelling, reading, sign language, etc. and that this can only be possible through multiple coding strategies. In effect, the advocates of total communication are calling for a "multilingual" individual. The present author knows of no research findings or psycholinguistic theories that would indicate that multiple coding is not possible. Moulton and Beasley state that "it is possible that hearing-impaired subjects may be capable of switching codes and that the coding system used varies with varying communication situations." Such a possibility could in part explain the excellent speech *and* manual communication skills of many deaf individuals.

Premise IV

Speech and manual forms of communication are not mutually exclusive. The present writer was trained as an oralist and spent many years teaching in what is reputed to be one of the better oral programs. He is well aware that sign language is often criticized as being such an efficient communication tool that its use tends to discourage other perhaps more "desirable" methods of communication, such as speech, speechreading, and residual hearing. The bulk of the research, however, indicates little if any, difference between the speech of deaf children trained in oral and total communication programs (Moores, 1971, 1978, and Vernon and Koh, 1970), and the experience of this author has been the same. From the previous section of this chapter on common speech problems of the deaf, it should be obvious that a statement of "no difference" between the speech of children in oral and total communication programs probably means that the speech is "equally bad" in both settings. It would seem that in any school for the deaf, regardless of philosophy, a normal curve exists relative to speaking ability. That is, a few children have "good" speech, the majority have speech that is somewhat intelligible, and a few have little or no speech skills. In some oral programs, especially the private schools, a high degree of selectivity plus a high "attrition rate" assures that the program graduates have better than average speech skills. The speech pathologist should realize that the selectivity and attrition rate of such programs may have as much to do with the relatively better speech skills as does the school's teaching philosophy and methods. The writer has often wondered what would happen if a total communication program could establish an initial screening program such that they admitted only those children whose parents could provide an optimal total communication atmosphere in the home and then to retain only those children who continued to progress in speech, language, sign language, etc.

It is often charged that speech is often given such cursory attention in total communication programs that the schools resemble the old manual programs of the last century. Sadly, there is probably a great deal of truth in this, and it may in part explain the poor speech of some deaf individuals. It may well be that if speech is not encouraged, especially during the younger years, the child develops a coding system that does *not* include acoustic or speech motor features and speech training then becomes extremely difficult. Most administrators of total communication programs are aware (if only on an intuitive level) of the dangers of singular coding strategies and constantly encourage parents and teachers to promote the use of speech.

The belief that sign language precludes speech has often led to the assumption that it is best to begin the child's preschool and elementary training in the oral or aural mode and then to hold total communication in reserve, to be used if the child fails to develop oral and auditory skills. When presented with such an argument, the speech pathologist should remember that the early years are of primary importance to language development and that to gamble that audition and speechreading will be sufficient for language development is just that, a gamble. Contemporary literature, on the other hand, indicates that when deaf children are presented with sign language that corresponds to English, language develops along normal lines (Brasel and Quigley, 1977; Costello, 1972; and Raffin, 1976).

Premise V

The deaf child's speech difficulty is primarily phonemic in nature. That is, the primary problem would appear to be related to the lack of concept development. Due to the limited input from the auditory channel, the child has difficulty in developing (extracting) correct images of the distinctive features of the language, such as voicing, frication, posterior place of articulation features (palatal, linguavelar, linguaalveolar) and the suprasegmental features relating to pitch, loudness, stress, and juncture. Even when such features are acquired, the deaf child will have problems learning the rules governing correct feature usage (See Chapter 1). While some children have neurological and orofacial defects that may limit production capability it is apparent that the primary deficits lie in the phonemic, not phonetic, realm.

As previously noted, the bulk of all speech therapy in programs for the deaf is phonetic in nature as are most speech development programs. Since, as noted in Chapter 6, the phonemic aspects of speech must precede the phonetic, considerable alteration of current speech development and correction programs is called for. Fortunately, the bulk of the approaches discussed in Chapter 6, though designed for use with hearing subjects, may be adapted for use with the deaf child. Some of these approaches and a few of their modifications for use with the hearing impaired are discussed below, but the speech pathologist with a bit of creativity should be able to take Chapter 6 and use it as a guide for the majority of his work with the deaf.

It will be recalled that the phonemic aspects of speech are developed through awareness of features or rules. For this, some discrimination training and a concomitant reliance on audition are usually considered necessary. The traditional approach to articulation therapy stresses a reopening of the servosystem and a reestablishment of auditory feedback until the speech problem is corrected and the individual can return to a kinesthetic feedback system. It is obvious that, for the hard of hearing at least, better auditory management should make it possible to use auditory feedback for speech correction. It occurs to this writer that the four steps of ear training (isolation, stimulation, identification, and discrimination) described by Van Riper (1972) would make an excellent guide for auditory training for the hard of hearing and some severe-profoundly deaf who can benefit from their residual hearing. For many deaf people, however, it may be that the auditory channel has little utility and some channel other than auditory must be used for the feedback process. Here, some visual form of feedback such as those electronic aids described by Pickett (1971) could be used. Mirror work and tactual techniques might also be tried.

The distinctive feature approach to speech correction is phonemic in nature and would also seem to rely on auditory training. The distinctive feature approach suggests that we select items for minimal pair contrasts in the auditory discrimination phase according to an analysis of consistent error patterns. Further, the distinctive feature approach calls for the use of some feature system such as that suggested by Chomsky and Halle (See Chapter 1). Note however, the abundance of features in the Chomsky and Halle system that would require hearing for their discrimination. Such an analysis of features may help the reader to understand why the speech of the hearing impaired is usually so affected. It should also convince the reader that some modification of the distinctive feature approach would be necessary for those individuals who cannot receive or utilize enough auditory input to handle the minimal pair contrasts used in phonemic training. When this occurs, some feedback system other than audition (tactual, visual, or kinesthetic) should be tried. Note however, that if the feature selected for contrast, such as plus or minus frication, is totally missing from the child's speech skills, it may well be that that feature is missing simply because it was never heard. When this is the case, considerable effort may be needed to first give the child the phonemic concept of the feature and then to help the child generalize that feature to related phonemes. Such a task is obviously different from that faced by the normal child who can hear the feature and who may have the feature already developed in some phonemes.

When, through auditory training or the use of compensatory feedback systems, the child realizes the value of speech, attempts to use speech to communicate, has developed a phonemic basis for speech, and has sufficient language to cooperate in the remediation program, the phonetic aspects of speech correction may begin. Any attempts to correct the motoric aspects of speech prior to this would only frustrate the child and be a waste of time better spent on other things. It does no good to teach a child how to produce speech sounds if the child has no concept of the connection between speech and language. Once again, the traditional approach to speech correction described in Chapter 6 contains many ideas that can readily be adapted to the deaf. In fact, the therapy steps outlined by Van Riper would probably work well with most hearing impaired individuals as long as the phonemic aspects of speech were intact before the phonetic aspects were stressed.

This writer is most impressed with the McDonald approach to phonetic speech correction (See Chapter 6). Note that McDonald stresses the use of correct tactile and kinesthetic images associated with accurate production and that the tactile and kinesthetic sensory modalities are very appropriate for instructional input to the deaf and hard of hearing. Also, McDonald states that the *syllable* is the basic unit of speech production and discourages the use of isolated phoneme drill. It will be recalled that it is the present author's opinion that many of the common speech problems of the deaf are directly related to an overemphasis of the use of isolated phonemes in the teaching situation. While some production training is undoubtedly needed in order to reinforce feature concepts and to provide the child with vital feedback references for production accuracy, isolated phoneme drills will not accomplish the goal of improved speech intelligibility. Speech therapy should aim at developing correct *natural* production in a variety of phonetic and linguistic contexts.

This writer must take some exception, however, to McDonald's recommendations of nonsense syllables, words, and sentences. The deaf child's lack of adequate exposure to English make nonsense syllables, words, and sentences confusing and are a waste of valuable time. Especially in words and sentences, it is just as easy for the speech clinician to use meaningful materials for speech activities that would then contribute to language growth.

Premise VI

When possible, speech therapy should be so structured as to promote normal language and conversation skills. All too often, the therapy session is seen by the deaf child as something removed from reality, and having little practical utility. When the speech clinician spends the bulk of a therapy session on repetitions of "bee-ba-boo" drills, the child may well ask "why—why—why?" All too often the educational programs for the deaf make a drastic separation between speech and language habilitation and this is unfortunate. Kretschmer and Kretschmer (1978) do an excellent job of pointing out that language is more than semantics, syntax, and vocabulary and they strongly suggest that teachers of the deaf should pay more attention to the pragmatic and conversational aspects of language. This suggests that therapy should, as soon as possible, focus on the conversational level and the meaningful expression of ideas rather than on drills with isolated phonemes or nonsense syllables, words or phrases. Too often, deaf children approach language in a word by word or sentence by sentence approach, resulting in problems in conversational, reading, and writing skills. The speech pathologist should not contribute to these problems by concentrating only on isolated aspects of language (phonemes, syllables, words, etc.) that have little utility by themselves.

The writer remembers conducting a speech class with a group of deaf teenagers and being concerned that there was little carry-over outside of the classroom. It seemed that the speech skills practiced in the classroom had little relevance to the lives that the children led when they left class. To rectify this situation, the writer arranged for a blind date party with a local public high school; sixty hearing teenagers volunteered to spend an evening with our deaf high school students in a dinner date situation. For several weeks the children in the writer's speech classes prepared for their "big night." We practiced speech and language related skills that we felt would be needed on a date with a hearing person and held many mock conversations and role playing situations. This all resulted in significant speech improvement that had meaning and obvious utility for the deaf teenagers.

SUMMARY

This chapter has described the hearing impaired population as being diverse in background and in speaking ability. The speech of the deaf has been depicted in rather bleak terms as being atypical in nearly all respects, but the speech pathologist should take heart in the fact that a good portion of the speech problems are probably the result of improper teaching practices rather than being directly caused by the hearing loss. Such speech problems caused by human error can only be alleviated by presenting more accurate information and demonstrating better techniques. It may be up to the speech pathologist to show us how to "build a better cabin" by using the blueprints available from contemporary research, theory, and techniques.

REFERENCES

Bargstadt, G. H., Hutchinson, J. M., and Nerbonne, M. A.: Learning visual correlates of fricative production by normal-hearing subjects: a preliminary evaluation of the video articulator. *J Speech Hear Disord, 63:*200-207, 1978.

Bender, R.: *The Conquest of Deafness.* Cleveland, Western Res Pr, 1960.

Black, J.: Speech Pathology for the Deaf. In Connor, L. (Ed.): *Speech for the Deaf Child: Knowledge and Use.* Washington, Alexander Graham Bell Association for the Deaf, 1971.

Boring, E. G.: *A History of Experimental Psychology.* New York, Appleton-Century-Crofts, 1950.

Brasel, K. and Quigley, S.: Influence of certain language and communication environments in early childhood on the development of language in deaf individuals. *J Speech Hear Res, 20:*95-107, 1977.

Brill, R., Merrill, E., and Frisina, D.: *Recommended Organizational Policies in the Education of the Deaf.* Washington, D.C., Conference of Executives of American Schools for the Deaf, 1973.

Calvert, D. R. and Silverman, R. S.: *Speech and Deafness.* Washington, D.C., Alexander Graham Bell Association for the Deaf, 1975.

Conrad, R.: Short-term memory processes in the deaf. *Brit J Psychol, 61:*179-195, 1970.

———: Some correlates of speech coding in the short-term memory of the deaf. *J Speech Hear Res, 16:*375-383, 1973.

Costello, E.: *Appraising Certain Linguistic Structures in the Receptive Sign Language Competence of Deaf Children.* Unpublished doctoral dissertation, Syracuse University, Syracuse, 1972.

Curtis, J. F.: Acoustics of speech production and nasalization. In Spriestersbach, C. D. and Sherman, D. (Eds.): *Cleft Palate and Communication.* New York, Acad Pr, 1968.

DiCarlo, L. M.: *The Deaf.* Englewood Cliffs, P-H, 1964.

Drum, Philip R.: How speech therapy feels. *Volta Rev, 65:*74-75, 1963.

Ewing, A. and Ewing, E.: *Teaching Deaf Children to Talk.* Washington, Volta Bureau, 1964.

Fraser, G.: Genetic approaches to the nasalogy of deafness. In Bergsma, D. (Ed.): *Clinical Delineation of Birth Defects.* Baltimore, Williams and Williams, 1971.

Frisina, R. (Chairman): Report of the Committee to Redefine Deaf and Hard of Hearing for Educational Purposes, 1974. (Mimeo)

Fry, B.: The role and primacy of the auditory channel in speech and language development. In Ross, M. and Giolas, T. (Eds.): *Auditory Management of Hearing-Impaired Children.* Baltimore, Univ Park, 1978.

Garnett, C. B.: *The World of Silence: A New Venture in Philosophy.* New York, Har-Row, 1967.

Groht, M.: *Natural Language for Deaf Children.* Washington, Alexander Graham Bell Association for the Deaf, 1958.

Heidinger, V. A.: *An Exploratory Study of Procedures for Improving Temporal Features in the Speech of Deaf Children.* Unpublished Doctoral Dissertation, Columbia University, 1972.

Holbrook, A. and Crawford, G. H.: Modification of vocal frequency and intensity in the speech of the deaf. *Volta Rev, 72:*492-497, 1970.

Holm, C.: Oral presentation at the first international colloquium on the verbotonal system. Primosten (Yugoslavia), January, 1970.

Hudgins, C. V.: A comparative study of the speech coordinations of deaf and normal subjects. *J Genet Psychol, 44:*3-48, 1934.

———: A study of respiration and speech. *Volta Rev, 38:*341-343, 1936.

———: Voice production and breath control in the speech of the deaf. *Am Ann Deaf, 82:*338-363, 1937.

Hyde, S. and Engle, D.: *The Potomac Program.* Beaverton, Dormac, 1977.

Johnson, D. M.: *Systematic Introduction to the Psychology of Thinking.* New York, Har-Row, 1972.

Jordan, I. K., Gustason, G., and Rosen, R.: Current communication trends at programs for the deaf. *Am Ann of the Deaf, 121:*527-532, 1976.

Konigsmark, B.: Syndromal approaches to the nasalogy of hereditary deafness. In Bergsma, D. (Ed.): *Clinical Delineation of Birth Defects.* Baltimore, Williams and Williams, 1971.

Kretschmer, R. and Kretschmer, L.: *Language Development and Intervention with the Hearing Impaired.* Baltimore, Univ Park, 1978.

Ling, D. and Ling, A.: *Aural Habilitation.* Washington, Alexander Graham Bell Association for the Deaf, 1978.

Ling, D.: *Speech and the Hearing-Impaired Child.* Washington, Alexander Graham Bell Association for the Deaf, 1976.

Locke, J. L.: Subvocal speech and speech. *ASHA, 12:*7-14, 1970.

McGinnis, M. A.: *Aphasic Children: Identification and Education by the Association Method.* Washington, Alexander Graham Bell Association for the Deaf. 1963.

Markides, A.: The speech of deaf and partially-hearing children with special reference to factors affecting intelligibility. *Brit J Disord Comm, 5:*126-140, 1970.

Mindel, E.: Studies on the deaf child. In Grinker, R. (Ed.): *Psychiatric Diagnosis, Therapy and Research on the Psychotic Deaf.* Washington, U.S. Department of Health, Education, and Welfare, Social and Rehabilitation Service, SRS-RSA-192-1971, 73-83, 1971.

Mindel, E. and Vernon, M.: *They Grow in Silence.* Silver Spring, Nat Ass Deaf, 1972.

Moores, D.: *Educating the Deaf: Psychology, Principles and Practices.* Boston, Houghton Mifflin, 1978.

————: *Recent Research in Manual Communication.* University of Minnesota Research, Development and Demonstration Center in Education of Handicapped Children, Occasional Paper, No. 7, 1971.

Moulton, R. D. and Beasley, D. S.: Verbal coding strategies used by hearing-impaired individuals. *J Speech Hear Res, 18:*559-570, 1975.

Nickerson, R.: Characteristics of the speech of deaf persons. *Volta Rev, 77:*342-361, 1975.

Pickett, J. M.: Speech science research and speech communication for the deaf. In Connor, L. E. (Ed.): *Speech for the Deaf Child.* Washington, Alexander Graham Bell Association for the Deaf, 1971.

Poole, I.: Genetic development in articulation of consonant sounds in speech. *Elementary Eng, 11:*159-161, 1934.

Proceedings of the International Conference on Oral Education of the Deaf, Washington, *Volta Bureau,* 1967.

Raffin, M.: *The Acquisition of Inflectional Morphemes by Deaf Children Using SEE Essential English.* Unpublished Doctoral Dissertation, University of Iowa, Iowa City, 1976.

Rawlings, B. and Trybus, R.: Personnel, facilities, and services available in schools and classes for hearing impaired children in the United States. *Am Ann Deaf, 123:*99-114, 1978.

Ross, M. and Giolas, T.: Introduction. In Ross, M. and Giolas, T. (Eds.): *Auditory Management of Hearing-Impaired Children.* Baltimore, Univ Park, 1978.

Scuri, D.: Restirazione e Fonazione nei Sardomuti. *Rassegna di Educazione e Fonetica Biologica, 14:*82-113, 1935.

Slobin, D.: *Psycholinguistics*. Glenview, Scott Foresman, 1971.

Smith, C. M.: *Residual Hearing and Speech Production in Deaf Children*. Unpublished Doctoral Dissertation, City University of New York, 1973.

Stinick, V., Rushmer, N., and Arpan, R.: *Parent-Infant Communication*. Beaverton, Dormac, 1978.

Templin, M.: *Certain Language Skills in Children*. Minneapolis, U of Minn, 1957.

————: Speech development in the young child: 3. the development of certain language skills in children. *J Speech Hear Disord, 17:*280-285, 1952.

Van Riper, C.: *Speech Correction: Principles and Methods*. Englewood Cliffs, P-H, 1972.

Vernon, M. and Koh, S.: Effects of oral preschool compared to manual communication on education and communication in deaf children. In Mindel, E. and Vernon, M.: *They Grow in Silence*. Silver Spring, Nat Ass Deaf, 1972.

Vorce, E.: *Teaching Speech to Deaf Children*. Washington, Alexander Graham Bell Association for the Deaf, 1974.

Wellman, B., Case, I., Mengert, I., and Bradbury, D.: *Speech Sounds of Young Children*. University of Iowa Studies in Child Welfare, *5, No. 2*, 1931.

Yale, C. A.: *Formation and Development of Elementary English Sounds*. Northampton, Clark School for the Deaf, 1938.

Index

287